Food Allergies and College:
Your Complete Planning Guide

Information, Recommendations and Insights

Food Allergies and College:
Your Complete Planning Guide

Information, Recommendations and Insights

JAN HANSON, M.A.

Cover, interior layout designed by Eric Wing, MetroCreate Studios, Mike Barry, East Coast Printing

Edited by Courtney Donahue-Taleporos

Library of Congress Cataloging-in-Publication Data

Hanson, Jan
 Food Allergies and College: Your Complete Planning Guide –
 Information, Recommendations and Insights / Jan Hanson

ISBN: 10: 1537552562

ISBN: 13: 978-1537552569

Library of Congress Control Number: 2016915105

CreateSpace Independent Publishing Platform, North Charleston, SC

DEDICATION

I dedicate this book to my two sons. Dan, you were ready for college, you knew what to do to safely manage your food allergies, and you did it with confidence. Will, you handled a new diagnosis of food allergy in stride, and didn't miss a beat. I am so proud of you both and of all of your accomplishments. I also dedicate this book to my husband, Mike, whose insights, belief in me, and constant encouragement for me to share my knowledge and experience with others, has kept me going throughout this project. You all have my sincere love and gratitude.

I also dedicate this book to college students with food allergies, and their families. You have been my motivation to write this book. Many of you have been successfully navigating this journey with energy and resilience and passion for what may seem like a very long time. For students who are newly diagnosed with a food allergy, know that you are not alone. As all of you get ready for this new phase of your life, stay the course, be prepared and know that you've got this!

Food Allergies and College:
Your Complete Planning Guide
Information, Recommendations and Insights

CONTENTS

CHAPTER TWO

FOOD ALLERGIES AND COLLEGE PLANNING: STRATEGIES AND RECOMMENDATIONS FOR STUDENTS AND PARENTS 35

CHAPTER THREE

WHAT WE CAN LEARN FROM STUDENTS WITH FOOD ALLERGIES WHO HAVE EXPERIENCED LIFE AT COLLEGE 87

CHAPTER FOUR

UNDERSTANDING THE LAWS THAT PROTECT COLLEGE STUDENTS WITH FOOD ALLERGIES 93

CHAPTER FIVE
FOOD ALLEGIES: A REFRESHER

ACKNOWLEDGEMENTS

I would like to sincerely thank everyone who contributed to my book. Your interest in improving the quality of life of college students with food allergies is respectfully acknowledged, and greatly appreciated. The information you have shared is invaluable.

Maria Laura Acebal, JD, Board Member, Food Allergy Research and Education (FARE), former CEO, Food Allergy and Anaphylaxis Network (now FARE).

Chelsea Black, Assistant Director, Office of Student Life/Housing Administration, The Ohio State University, Columbus, Ohio.

Joanne Clinch, MD, Clinical Director, Student Health Services, Wake Forest University, Winston-Salem, North Carolina.

Donna DeCosta, MD, Author, *A Little Bit Can Hurt.*

Nicholas Ditzler, College Student, University of Michigan, Ann Arbor, Michigan.

Lisa Eberhart, RD, LDN, CDE, Director of Nutrition and Wellness, North Carolina State University, Raleigh, North Carolina.

Tanner Elvidge, College Student, Northeastern University, Boston, Massachusetts.

Ethan Faust, College Student, Davidson College, Davidson, North Carolina.

Mackenzie Gannon, College Student, Ithaca College, Ithaca, New York.

Kristi Grim, National Programs Manager, Food Allergy Research and Education (FARE), McLean, Virginia.

Dan Hanson, Recent College Graduate, The George Washington University, Washington, DC.

Linda Herbert, Ph.D., Psychologist, Division of Allergy & Immunology, Children's National Health System, Washington, DC.

Kristie Orr, Ph.D., Director of Disability Services, Texas A&M University, College Station, Texas.

Scott Riccio, Senior Vice President of Education and Advocacy, Food Allergy Research and Education (FARE), McLean, Virginia.

Nancy Rotter, Ph.D., Pediatric Psychologist, Food Allergy Center, Massachusetts General Hospital, Boston, Massachusetts.

Kathleen Shannon, Recent College Graduate, North Carolina State University, Raleigh, North Carolina.

Lisa Stieb, RN, BSN, AE-C, Food Allergy Center, Massachusetts General Hospital, Boston, Massachusetts.

Anne Thompson, Co- Founder, Mothers of Children Having Allergies (MOCHA), Chicago, Illinois.

Megan Yee, College Student, Northwestern University, Evanston, Illinois.

I am honored to have had your assistance, and grateful to you all!

FOREWORD

College. Just the thought of a child reaching the age where preparations for college begin generates significant anxiety for all parents, and that anxiety is often magnified many fold for parents of children with life-threatening food allergies. According to a study released in 2013 by the Centers for Disease Control and Prevention, food allergies among children increased approximately 50% between 1997 and 2011. Data tells us that many of these children are not outgrowing those allergies, meaning that more and more of them are now heading off to college still dealing with their food allergy in addition to the myriad new challenges that college can bring. This means there are also an ever-growing number of parents dealing with a lot of worry for the safety of their college-bound, food-allergic children.

Unfortunately, until recently, there has not been a uniform set of best practice guidelines, nor consistent expert support for implementation of practices at the college and university level to keep students with food allergies safer and more included. In response to this need, FARE launched our College Food Allergy Program in January 2014 with the goal of developing a comprehensive program to improve the safety and quality of life for college students with food allergies. FARE partnered with the National Foundation for Celiac Awareness, the National Association of College & University Food Services, the Association on Higher Education and Disability, food allergy experts, and stakeholders including staff representatives from colleges and universities, as well as parents and students, to help determine needs, set goals and guide the direction of the program.

As a result of the hard work and expertise shared by these committed individuals and organizations, FARE released the "Pilot Guidelines for Managing Food Allergies in Higher Education" in 2015, and launched a pilot phase at 12 colleges and universities. In 2016, thanks to the hard work of our staff, volunteers and, and pilot schools, and the generosity of supporters, FARE is expanding our program to include 40 colleges and universities.

Jan's book brings to life many of the best practices, insights from expert contributors and stories illuminating the importance of a comprehensive and collaborative approach to support both students and staff at colleges and universities. The extensive information provided, including step-by-step recommendations for college planning, creates a framework which will empower college-bound students and their families. This approach, combined with Jan's personal and professional expertise and network of like-minded expert solution finders, makes this book such an important contribution to our community.

Jan Hanson, founder of her consulting company, Educating For Food Allergies, LLC (EFFA) has spent more than 25 years helping families, schools and colleges, and the entire community involved in helping care for those with food allergies. Jan has helped families through challenging situations, whether through prudent planning, education, or improvements in organizational policies, always with the approach of partnership and collaboration to find solutions.

Having worked as the Assistant Director of Residence Life at Simmons College, an educator and a mom with two children who went off to college with food allergies, Jan is perfectly suited to help build the bridges necessary to bring the entire college community together in support of better care and safer environments for students with food allergies. Any teenagers who are now or one day considering college, and their parents, as well as anyone who is involved with the support and care of these students, will benefit from reading and incorporating the knowledge and practices included in this valuable book.

Scott Riccio, Senior Vice President, Education and Advocacy
Food Allergy Research and Education (FARE)

PREFACE

From the Author

Going to college with a food allergy can present some unique considerations, and safety is often at the forefront. I know because I have two sons who went off to college with food allergies, one in 2005 and one in 2009. There were no books available at that time to help. We incorporated questions about how to handle food allergies into our discussions, and I am delighted to share that this challenge was successfully navigated!

For the past fifteen years I have worked as a food allergy educator helping students, families and school personnel throughout the United States manage food allergies. Years earlier, after receiving my graduate degree in Higher Education Administration, I worked as the Assistant Director of Residence Life at Simmons College. I lived on campus, working closely with the resident advisors and student government representatives. Because of my role as a college administrator, I know firsthand the kinds of issues that can arise in this setting.

I have written this book for those of you with food allergies who are ready to make plans for college, and your families who are helping and supporting you, so that I can assist you with your journey. My experiences, both personally and professionally, have put me in a unique position to make this sometimes overwhelming process a little easier.

Please use this guide in whatever way you feel will be most helpful – to learn new information to assist you in your planning, to reaffirm and review what you already know, or perhaps as a catalyst for your discussions. The information and recommendations I have outlined in this book are consistent with and in direct support of the guidance which Food Allergy Research and Education (FARE) offers to colleges and universities in their pilot College Food Allergy Program.

CHAPTER ONE

Food Allergies And College Offices:
A Description Of Services So You Know
What To Expect

"Education is all a matter of building bridges."
-Ralph Ellison, American Novelist and College Professor

If you are a junior in high school, then life is undoubtedly very busy. You are probably juggling a full load of classes, as well as several extracurricular activities. Social engagements may be taking up a great deal of your time, and may include everything from informal parties with friends, to plans for big events like the Junior Prom. If going to college after graduation is in your future, then this year will be filled with activities geared toward making this goal a reality. Preparing for and taking the SATs and related exams is a major focus, as is the process of figuring out which colleges or universities you will pursue. Meetings with your guidance counselor and discussions with your parents will help you to consider factors such as preferences you may have about academic programs available, geographic locations and the size of the college you'd like to attend. Many students and their families will travel to visit college campuses to help "get a feeling" for the school. This is an exciting time!

If you are a high school junior with food allergies who is making plans for college, there is another important factor for you to consider:

WILL THE COLLEGE ADEQUATELY ACCOMMODATE AND
MAKE ARRANGEMENTS FOR ME TO ATTEND SAFELY WITH
FOOD ALLERGIES?

While academic programs and class offerings may be a starting point in your college search, why should the question of how a college manages food allergies on campus be a variable worth considering? The information in this chapter will help make clear why this should be an important consideration, and will help you understand what to look for as you evaluate how well each institution is managing this task. The end result: you'll be able to make more informed decisions, so that you can determine what schools would be the "best fit" for you.

Background

We know that when you have a food allergy, coming into contact with your allergen can happen in a variety of ways and in virtually all settings and locations. This is not new information. At college, you'll need to navigate food and beverages not only in the dining halls, but also in the residence halls and across campus. The question is: what are colleges and universities doing to help the growing number of students coming to campus with food allergies, food restrictions or celiac disease? The answer depends on the college or university. Progress is being made in this area, however, and more and more institutions of higher education are providing the services needed for their students with food allergies and food restrictions to be able to attend school more safely.

Unfortunately, there is still no standard, or universally accepted approach or common understanding of how food allergies should be managed on college campuses. You will find there is considerable variability in what each college is doing, regardless of the institution's size, or whether it is public or private. To put it simply, some schools are much better at having procedures in place that meet the needs of their student population with food allergies and food restrictions, while others are not.

Research about what practices are being implemented by institutions of higher education to accommodate the needs of students with food allergies and food intolerances is, to date, quite limited. In fact, information on this topic is so lacking that it appears only two studies have been published which investigated food allergy management procedures at colleges and universities, and these focused only on university dining services. The findings of these two studies are included in the Supplemental Materials found at the end of this chapter. What is happening, or not happening, in residence halls and other locations on campus to reduce allergen exposure, for the most part, will depend on the individual college or university.

It will be up to you to determine what is being done to manage students' food allergies on each of the campuses that you have an interest, and based on this assessment, whether you believe you would be able to live and eat safely at that college or university. There are four college administrative offices you need to be familiar with to help you do this:

Housing/Residence Life, Dining Services, Health Services and Disability Services.

These are the four offices that you should investigate in order to find out what they are doing, and what they would be willing to do, for you to attend college safely.

In Part One of this chapter I describe the role and responsibilities of each of these four college offices, and after each description, I've included what is currently being practiced in randomly selected colleges in the U.S. In Part Two, I've outlined what are considered "best practices" of these four campus offices, so that you can better evaluate the services offered at the colleges you investigate.

As you begin to research schools, be aware that some institutions will have a fair amount of information on their website to give you an idea of what practices are being implemented by these four college offices to meet the special needs of their students with dietary restrictions, while others are much more limited in the information they choose to post online.

PART ONE: DESCRIPTION OF COLLEGE ADMINISTRATIVE OFFICES

Let's get started so that you will have a good understanding of the role and function of these four campus offices. After each campus office description, I've included examples of services, either directly, or indirectly, related to food allergies that I found on the websites of randomly selected colleges and universities across the country. In this way, you'll have an idea of the variability of what may be available. A word of caution: although a web search can provide you with some information, it's always a good idea to contact these offices directly to get the most up-to-date and complete information about the services each institution offers.

Please Note: The abbreviated descriptions of campus services highlighted in Part One are based on information posted on each of the institution's websites *at the time of this book's publication*.

1. **DISABILITY SERVICES OFFICE**

The main purpose and goal of the college's Disability Services Office should be to respond effectively to the special needs of its students with a disability, including those with a food allergy or celiac disease. Life-threatening food allergies and severe food restrictions generally meet the criteria and legal definition of a disability (see Chapter Four for more information on civil rights laws). The Disability Services Office should ensure that all of its students who have a disability are not discriminated against in any way, and are provided reasonable and appropriate accommodations so that they may have full access to campus programs. The name of this office varies from school to school, and you may find it listed under many titles, including the Office of Accessible Education, or the Student and Employee Accessibility Services Office, for example.

When a student with a disability contacts the Disability Office and requests that accommodations be provided by the college to allow for his or her safe participation, it is common practice for this office to ask for documentation of the disability. For a student with a life-threatening food allergy, for example, this documentation is typically a doctor's statement which identifies the student as having this health diagnosis. Paperwork and forms required by the college in order to evaluate and determine if special services will be provided, should be given to the student, with the request that they be completed and submitted back to the institution within set deadlines. Once documentation and related information has been received, the institution will decide if the health diagnosis constitutes a disability under the Americans with Disabilities Act (ADA). If it is determined that this is the case, then appropriate modifications to the college's programs and services should be made for the student.

Information about how you should begin this process and access the required forms may be found on the Disability Office's page of the school's website. As noted earlier, differences exist from one college to another with regard to the information posted online. For some schools, instructions may be very detailed, and include staff names, titles and contact information, procedures to follow for disability documentation, including deadlines that must be met with links provided to access the necessary forms, and examples given of reasonable accommodations for campus dining and housing. Web page content for other college disability offices can be very basic, and not as user-friendly as you might like.

Although every college or university has the right to establish its own requirements for disability documentation procedures, all institutions of higher education must be in compliance with Section 504 of the Rehabilitation Act of 1973 and The Americans with Disabilities Act (ADA), based on either Title II or Title III. The only exception to this legal obligation would be a religious institution that does not receive any federal funding. (See Chapter Four for more information.)

Examples of College Disability Services

Dickinson College, Carlisle, Pennsylvania

Office of Disability Services (ODS). Information about Dietary Accommodations on the ODS webpage at Dickinson College indicates that although all residential students are required to purchase a meal plan, Dickinson College has established procedures to ensure that students with a documented disability will have access to "reasonable on-campus dietary accommodations." Examples of current dietary accommodations offered include, "gluten-free and lactose-free options, vegan diets, a Star-K-certified kosher kitchen, and the ability to request alternative meals if necessitated by a medical condition." Food allergy is not specifically referenced.

Specific information about possible housing accommodations for students with food allergies is not listed.

Ohio State University, Columbus, Ohio

Office of Student Life Disability Services. The list of "Qualifying Conditions" posted on the Disability Service's website does not specifically include "food allergy." It is stated in bold print that the list provided is not comprehensive.

For information posted online about "Housing/Dining Accommodations", it states that "Students who ONLY need housing or dining do not need to register with Disability Services." For dining accommodations, the information provided is limited, and states that there are "alternative dining options located in dining facilities throughout the campus", and that these locations have signs placed near foods served regarding "some food allergies and restrictions such as gluten free, peanut free, and dairy free."

You are instructed to contact the Assistant Director of Nutrition for more information, and a name, telephone number and email address are provided.

2. DINING SERVICES OFFICE

It is the responsibility of Dining Services to purchase, prepare and serve food on campus for breakfast, lunch and dinner that meets federal and state food safety codes. Colleges have a multitude of different venues where students may eat, ranging from campus dining halls, dining rooms located in residence halls, university coffee shops, convenience stores, snack kiosks, events that are catered, and informal parties or gatherings, for example. The knowledge of dining services employees, and their response to the needs of their student population with food allergies and food restrictions, varies from college to college. For example, some college dining halls will have ingredient lists clearly posted, including food allergens present in foods served, while other institutions do not provide this kind of information. Some university dining staff are educated about food allergies and trained in prevention of allergen exposure, while this is not the case at others. Most colleges and universities will have a dining hall manager present in the dining hall when meals are being served. Many campus dining services will also have a registered dietitian available to assist students in making health and safe food choices.

Examples of College Dining Services

Brown University, Providence, Rhode Island

Students who need special dietary accommodations who are admitted to Brown University must register with the Student and Employee Accessibility Services Office at least three weeks before coming to campus, and complete all required paperwork. It is the student's responsibility to meet with the school's Registered Dietitian, and then a reasonable accommodation plan will be developed for the student. The campus dining service's web page has a "Nutrition and Allergies" link, which lists dietary forms and gives information about nut-free salad bars and alternative foods to anything containing peanuts and nuts. Retail food sites on campus may have foods containing peanuts, tree nuts and other allergens, and students with food allergies are instructed to use caution with these vendors.

Stanford University, Stanford, California

At Stanford, the Ricker Dining room on campus has been designated as a "Peanut-Sensitive Environment", and is lauded as the first facility of this kind in the nation. Peanut products are not prepared or served by food service personnel here, and students may not bring any food of their own into Ricker Dining Room. Stanford University also offers a Gluten-Free MicroKitchen located in the Arrillaga Family Dining Commons.

Saint Anselm College, Manchester, New Hampshire

St. Anselm College has a written policy statement: *Saint Anselm Policy on Food Allergy Accommodations for Students.* The policy includes: a commitment to allergen risk reduction, requirements for food service staff to be trained in food allergy awareness, and requirements for labeling food items that contain allergenic ingredients. The policy states that students need to inform the College of their diagnosis and need for special dietary requests. Procedures within the policy also require food-allergic students to provide medical documentation to the Director of Health Services, for the completion of a form to allow for this information to be shared with the Director of Dining Services, and the requirement that the student meet personally with the Dining Service Director to tour the kitchen and learn about safe food options. An individual plan is developed to meet each student's needs.

Liberty University, Lynchburg, Virginia

Liberty University, which uses Sodexo as its dining service food supplier, has adopted Sodexo's *Simple Servings* Program. With this program, seven of the "Top Eight" food allergens (milk, eggs, soy, tree nuts, peanuts, shellfish, and wheat), as well as gluten, are eliminated from all foods being served. In addition, it is Liberty University's philosophy and practice not to single out students with food allergies in the dining hall.

NOTE: The *Simple Servings* Program offered by Sodexo is used at more than 100 colleges and universities across the country.

Bucknell, University, Lewisburg, Pennsylvania

Bucknell University has a page on its website titled: Dining and Food Allergy Accommodations. An overview of the campus dining services is given, including information about the *EatWell* program, which is an online tool designed to allow students to view nutritional information and filter food choices by allergens. The site describes the process and timeline expected for students to request special dietary accommodations, and indicates that the University's registered dietitian can meet with the student to review menu options and assist the process of making safe food selections.

3. HOUSING/RESIDENCE LIFE OFFICE

The primary functions of this office are twofold:

> 1.) To have procedures in place to allow for room assignments to be made for the student population who seek housing, based on living options available, and that take into account student profiles, preferences and needs, and

> 2.) To address residence life issues and respond adequately to the needs of its resident students, once they have moved in.

Once you have been accepted to a college or university, the Housing Office will ask you to complete and return forms that typically ask for information about you, such as personality traits, sleeping habits, as well as room preferences. You should know that living arrangement options are not the same at every college and university. Dormitories may have single rooms, doubles, triples, and even quads. The rooms with more occupants typically will have a common area, in addition to the bedrooms. Some rooms will have a semi-private bathroom for roommates to share. Some residence halls have a kitchen facility for the students to use, while others do not. Many colleges have apartment-style living options, both on, and off-campus, with a private kitchen for the residents of that apartment. You will find that some schools have a dedicated dining facility located in the residence hall for students to take their meals. You should also be aware that colleges will differ in the type of living arrangement offered to first year students, versus those which may be made available to upperclassmen.

Most, if not all, colleges and universities have Resident Advisor (RA) programs. The Residence Life Office is responsible for selecting and training these student Resident Advisors, and will assign them to floors within each residence hall. Some of these RAs receive education about food allergies and allergic reactions, while others do not. It is also possible to find colleges that assign an adult to live in the residence hall, often with a title similar to "Resident Director" or "Head Resident" who have specific responsibilities, such as supervising the RAs living in their residential building.

You Should Know: On some college campuses you may find only one office which is listed as either the Housing Office, or the Residence Life Office. In these cases, services relative to both housing and residence life are addressed under one roof.

Examples of College Housing Office Services

Rutgers University, New Brunswick, New Jersey

Rutgers University has a link on its website listed as: Housing for Students with Disabilities. Information is offered here about what criteria is used to determine a disability, and eligibility for services. Examples of accommodations which Rutgers will generally "NOT approve" for an accommodation includes a "Request for single living accommodations by students with asthma or allergies."

University of Massachusetts, Amherst, Massachusetts

Students may submit a Room Preference Application to the Residence Life Student Services Office at the University of Massachusetts. For accommodation requests that are based on medical reasons, you are instructed to contact the campus Disability Office, and a link and telephone number are included. Several examples of possible medical accommodations are listed on the Disability Office webpage, including assigning a student with severe allergies to a room that doesn't have a carpet. Accommodations for a student with severe *food* allergies are not included on this list.

4. <u>HEALTH SERVICES OFFICE</u>

The Health Services Office coordinates student health forms and information, and provides, and/or coordinates, health services on campus, including health management, non-emergency care and emergency response.

Most, but not all, colleges and universities have some type of health clinic available directly on campus. Health Service facilities will vary, however, from one institution to another, in terms of size, personnel and hours of operation. Some colleges will have small day clinics, others will have clinics equipped with beds for overnight stays to address minor medical concerns, and some larger universities will have a full-service teaching hospital located directly on campus.   Smaller schools may not have a doctor staffed at the clinic, but will likely have physicians available for referral.

Services offered at each campus health clinic will also vary. While most clinics will offer basic healthcare services, not all will provide counseling services or allergy shots, for example. You should also be aware that not all campus clinics are open 24 hours, on the weekends or on holidays. Larger universities may have an on-campus pharmacy, while this may not be a feature available at smaller institutions.

Campus emergency response capabilities also vary greatly from one college to another. For example, some schools train their campus police and/or students as the first responders to a medical emergency, while other campuses have professional emergency medical technicians (EMTs) and/or paramedics on staff for these situations. It is important to understand that not all emergency responders will have access to, or are trained and able to give epinephrine, should it be required. While all paramedics are trained to administer epinephrine, only some EMTs will have the training and ability to do so, and this will depend on state law.

The distance from campus to a full-service hospital, should it be required, will also differ, in some instances significantly, from one institution to another. In some instances, the campus first responders may call the local hospital ambulance to campus to transport a student back to the hospital.

Examples of Campus Health Services

Lehigh University, Bethlehem, Pennsylvania

Services provided at the Health Center include acute and routine care for students, including counseling services. Several pharmacies are within walking distance of the campus. The Health Center is closed after 4:30pm, Monday through Friday, and is closed on Sundays.

The Lehigh Emergency Medical Services, which is a Quick Response Service, offers basic life- support services, 24/7, and is staffed by student volunteers who are certified EMTs. All first responders are trained in EpiPen® administration, and the Quick Response vehicle carries epinephrine. First responders will assess the emergency, and call for the town EMS and an ambulance, if required.

Skidmore College, Saratoga Springs, New York

The Health Center located on the Skidmore College campus provides preventive and routine health care. It is staffed by nurse practitioners, registered nurses, two part-time physicians, and a registered dietitian. The Health Center is not equipped to administer allergy shots. A separate Counseling Center is located on campus.

The Skidmore College Emergency Medical Services team is comprised entirely of student volunteers who are all New York state certified at the EMT level, or higher. They are the first responders on campus and work closely with the local hospital emergency department.

NOTE: Examples of college and university programs and features included in Part One of this chapter have been abbreviated. Please go directly onto the website of the colleges or universities you are interested in for more information about services offered and the process for making specific arrangements and accommodation requests.

PART TWO: EXAMPLES OF "BEST SERVICES"

"The major test of a modern university is how wisely and how quickly it adjusts to important new possibilities."

-Clark Kerr
College Professor, 12th President, University of California

The College or University

In Part Two of this chapter, I'll review what are considered to be "best services" by colleges and universities, in their efforts to manage food allergies on campus. This will assist you in determining which schools you are investigating may best respond to your needs and preferences. In general, best service means that the college or university is prepared to meet the needs of its growing population of students with food allergies and celiac disease. These schools should have a formal, written policy which includes specific protocols and procedures to facilitate the process to:

1.) Determine a student's eligibility for protection under the ADA and Section 504, and

2.) Determine what accommodations/modifications will be made for each eligible student.

Specifically, it should:

- Establish standard operating procedures in all relevant areas of the college (*e.g.* Disability, Housing, Residence Life, Dining and Health), that allow for and promote a coordinated and collaborative effort between college offices.

- Provide guidance and training to university employees on how certain tasks should be performed in an effort to reduce food allergen exposure.

- Provide specific direction on emergency response.

- Provide relevant information on the homepage of the university website directing students with disabilities to the appropriate links.

The Association on Higher Education and Disability® (AHEAD), and the FARE College Pilot Program are valuable resources which offer guidance to these institutions to establish best service standards for policies regarding their students with disabilities.

1. <u>DISABILITY SERVICES OFFICE</u>

Best service in a college Disability Office means that there should be a written policy that addresses the college's commitment to effectively meet the needs of its students with disabilities, including those with food allergies. Staff in this office should be fully aware that the U.S. Department of Justice, in a settlement agreement with Lesley University in 2012, determined that some individuals with food allergy and celiac disease "have a disability as defined by the ADA, particularly those with more significant or severe responses to certain foods." (More information about this landmark settlement agreement can be found in Chapter Four.)

Clear information should be provided by staff which enables you to understand the process required to request formal accommodations. In addition, the Disability Office's page of the college's website should have information posted, with keywords listed that will help you find step-by-step guidance about the process you will need to follow. Once required paperwork has been submitted, your eligibility for services should be evaluated and you should be notified, in writing, about the college's decision as to whether or not your diagnosis of food allergy, celiac disease or other health diagnosis of a severe food restriction has been determined to meet the definition of a disability. Reasonable accommodations the college determines are necessary in order for you to be able to have full access to your academic program should be provided to you in writing, as well. The Disability Office can also play an important role in assisting you with other campus offices if you've been unable to fulfill academic obligations, such as missing a class or a test, for example, if the reason was due to a doctor's appointment, emergency care or other medical reason related to your health diagnosis.

The entire process for evaluation and the provision of services and accommodations should be completed in a timely way.

Best services should include:

- Helping you to understand your rights and readily answering any and all questions you may have.

- Providing you:

  - ➢ Names, titles, and telephone numbers of college staff you will need to contact,
  - ➢ Requirements the college has for you to document your food allergy,
  - ➢ An outline of the step-by-step procedures for you to follow,
  - ➢ Any forms you will need to complete, and
  - ➢ The timeline recommended (*e.g.* when you should start this process) and deadlines you must meet to submit required information.

- Making decisions regarding the need for modifications for a student on a case-by-case basis; these decisions should be independent of what has been done, or hasn't been done, at the institution before.

- Determining reasonable accommodations that are necessary for you to attend the college safely and achieve your academic goals. An example would be exemption from mandatory meal plans, if required.

- Coordinating your health plan with other departments and offices, such as Housing/Residence Life and Dining Services, for example.

- Keeping information about you and your disability confidential, and at the same time sharing this information and your health plan with appropriate personnel in the college's other offices where you will be receiving accommodations.

- Having a grievance process in place to address situations if you disagree with a decision made by the Disability Office regarding an accommodation in your health plan.

Insight: **Kristie Orr, Ph.D., Director of Disability Services,**
Texas A&M University

When visiting colleges, it is important to visit with the Disability Services office on campus. This office may be known by other names such as the Disability Resource Center, Accessibility Center, Student Disability Services, *etc.* Searching the college website for the office that works with students with disabilities should help you to locate this resource. The role of these offices is to promote access for students with disabilities by educating others on campus and determining appropriate academic adjustments. These offices can usually visit with students before they make their decision about which college to attend and provide information about adjustments (also known as accommodations) that can be made given the student's specific disabilities. Students can call and talk to a Disability Services staff member on the phone or visit the campus and meet with someone in order to determine what kind of accommodations might be appropriate and how to access those accommodations.

Once a student has decided to attend a specific college or university, they should check with the Disability Services office to determine how to register for services. Typically, a student meets with a staff member to talk about their needs and provides documentation in the form of a letter from their physician indicating the impact of their allergy and the specific allergies of that student. The student and staff member participate in an interactive process to determine how to best meet that student's needs and the staff member provides a letter to the student with the accommodations listed and/or communicates directly with the other offices that need to be informed (*i.e.,* housing, dining services).

Accommodations are determined on a case-by-case basis depending on the specific student's needs. Accommodations may include being placed in a residence hall near a specific dining facility that is best equipped to meet the student's needs, being in a single room or placed with a roommate that the student knows who agrees to abstain from having the student's allergens in the residence hall room, having a residence hall room with a private kitchen, being placed on a modified or reduced meal plan, or other accommodations that meet the student's needs. These accommodations are communicated to the housing office and/or dining services as appropriate and the Disability Services staff member is available to assist if there are concerns that come up with the university's ability to meet the student's needs.

Students are encouraged to contact their coordinator or counselor in the Disability Services office if they feel that their needs are not being met so that the Disability Services office can help advocate and problem-solve in order to make sure that the college or university is providing equal access for students with disabilities.

2. DINING SERVICES OFFICE

College campus food service operations must ensure that safe foods are served to their food-allergic patrons for meals at breakfast, lunch and dinner, accurate information is provided about the ingredients of foods being served, and staff is adequately trained. Without the provision of these three basic standards, students with food allergies will be at an increased risk for exposure to one of their food allergens, and experiencing an allergic reaction and anaphylaxis.

Best services should include:

- Developing and implementing policies and procedures specific to the type of food venues offered on campus, such as a dining hall, convenience store, food kiosk and catering.

- Maintaining allergen-control practices to avoid the possibility of cross-contact, such as:

  ➢ Using dedicated equipment for allergen-free food preparation,
  ➢ Assigning designated allergen-free food surfaces and areas for food preparation used by dining service cooks, and
  ➢ Providing dedicated allergen-safe food stations.

- When required, providing access to allergen-safe areas to prepare food given to students with food allergies or celiac disease. This could be a dedicated area in the dining hall kitchen, or a separate area entirely for this purpose.

- Providing students with information and access to safe food choices, such as:

  - ➤ The ability to pre-order meals, and
  - ➤ Offering meals that eliminate the top eight food allergens.

- Providing information about ingredients of foods served by utilizing one or more of the following strategies:

  - ➤ Posting clear ingredient labels of foods being served,
  - ➤ Providing food ingredient information related to the various campus dining venues on the college website's dining services page, and
  - ➤ Through consultation with the school's registered dietician, chef and/or dining hall manager.

- Dining Hall Services should meet the requirements of US Food Code 2013, such as making sure both full and part-time employees are able to identify the eight major food allergens, for example. Front-line staff must be prepared to accurately answer questions about ingredients of the foods they are serving.

You Should Know: There are resources to help college and university dining services in their efforts to provide a safer dining experience for their students and patrons with food allergies and restrictions.

■ The International Association of Food Protection provides icons that can be clearly posted to indicate ingredients of foods that contain, or potentially contain, food allergens.

■ A menu-labeling document developed by the U.S. Food and Drug Administration (FDA) offers guidance for foodservice directors in their efforts to provide accurate information.
(www.fda.gov/RegulatoryInformation/Guidances/default.htm.)

■ CBORD, a company that provides food and nutrition management, has online software known as NetNutrition® which is used by some colleges and universities. According to the CBORD website, this software enables students to "view menu offerings, identify possible allergens or food intolerances, select diet preferences, and analyze the nutritional content of meals."

■ Sodexo, a food service company used by many colleges and universities, offers the "Simple Servings Program", which includes a food station that eliminates gluten and seven of the Top Eight food allergens (milk, eggs, wheat, soy, shellfish, peanuts and tree nuts) in a way that does not isolate students with food allergies from the dining hall experience.

■ MenuTrinfo® provides accurate nutritional information to menu labeling for compliance with FDA regulations. AllerTrainU, offered by MenuTrinfo LLC, is a 90-minute training program designed for people who serve food in a college or university. Certification is given upon successful completion of this training. It is the only allergy training specific to university food service on the market, as of this book's publication date. A great resource provided by MenuTrinfo, LLC is an interactive map of the United States that indicates, by state, which colleges and universities have received AllerTrainU training. For more information you can go to their website at: http://allertrain.com/allertrained-college-and-universities/.

Note: When you speak with staff in College Dining Services, you can ask them if they use any of the resources mentioned.

Insight: **Lisa Eberhart, RD, LDN, CDE, Director of Nutrition and Wellness, North Carolina State University**

When you go away to college, food is an important part of the "community" on campus. As a student you want to be able to eat with your friends and have foods you enjoy. Making a decision on the college you will attend shouldn't be all about food and allergies, but it is part of the equation. You want to be part of the college community and that includes eating on campus.

The number one question to ask an institution of higher learning is, do you know what is in your food? The second question should be, how is this communicated to the customer? If the school cannot do these two things effectively then you won't be able to make educated and safe menu decisions. Some of the challenges that you may face when eating away from home at a restaurant, are the same when eating at a big institution.

When looking for a good fit you will need to know what the philosophy of the school is and if they are committed to helping you navigate their food system in a safe manner. Take a look at the school, go visit, is there anything you can eat?

At North Carolina State we are committed to helping the student with food allergies or intolerances have a normal college experience. This means being able to safely eat on campus and having as many choices as possible. We have everything analyzed down to the ingredient level so students can look at the complete ingredient list of any menu item on campus. The student needs to be able to glance at a digital menu board and identify allergens or quickly reference the mobile app. The student should be able to access an I-pad display or the website to get complete ingredient lists. If the school you are considering doesn't have this information at your fingertips, eating on campus will be a challenge.

The school should also support you emotionally and socially. Does the school have an allergy support group and a way to communicate with you about events on campus when it comes to allergies? At NC State we have a system where we email students, who self-identify as having an allergy or intolerance, about upcoming events, menu changes and tips. We have an allergy blogger who looks at all dining events and advises students on the upcoming special meal. We also offer allergy ambassadors who will give you peer to peer advice and tours of the dining facilities, mainly giving you some insight on how they handled their allergies on campus.

The school should also make sure you know what your responsibilities are when it comes to managing your allergies on campus. They should be very clear on their responsibilities too. What kind of training do they do with their staff and what do they do to minimize cross contact issues? Make sure the school has a registered dietitian that can help you with any food issues. I would advise that you chat with chefs and managers when visiting the school and let them know of your food issue. If they seem receptive and helpful that is a positive sign. Once you know the school understands food allergies and is responsive to students with allergies and intolerances you can make an educated choice about what school to attend.

3. HOUSING/RESIDENCE LIFE OFFICE

The Housing/Residence Life Office should have procedures in place to allow for room assignments to be made for their student population that take into account student profiles, preferences and needs, including those with food allergies, and based on housing options available. Housing forms should be designed to allow for sufficient information to be shared and reasonable requests to be made. Best services mean that Resident Advisors, as well as Resident Directors, should be trained to recognize and respond to the needs of students on their floors and in their residence halls, including those with food allergies, so that all students may participate safely in planned activities.

In addition, this office should work collaboratively with the Admissions Office, as well as the Student Activities or Student Affairs Office, in the planning and execution of planned campus activities, such as Freshmen Orientation, for example.

Best services should include:

- Providing accommodations for living arrangements which enable their student population with life-threatening allergies to live safely. Whether the student with this disability is a first-year student should not influence these decisions.

- Training and educating Residence staff, such as Resident Advisors or adult "Head Residents" that includes information about the health condition of food allergies and allergic reactions/anaphylaxis, and emergency procedures.

- Providing education about food allergies to students and student organizations on campus, such as those responsible for giving campus tours, incoming student orientation activities and Greek Life, for examples.

Insight: **Chelsea Black, Assistant Director, Office of Student Life/Housing Administration, The Ohio State University**

At The Ohio State University, students have the opportunity to identify any food allergies when completing their housing contracts. They can also designate on the contract if they are in need of special accommodations due to their allergies. Depending on the need, the student's assignment may be to a single room (*i.e.*, in the case of a peanut allergy) or to a room with access to a kitchen if that will afford them the best opportunity to manage their allergies.

The relationship between University Housing, Dining Services and Disability Services is a collaborative one. In the event that the student or parent reaches out to Disability Services or Dining Services prior to contacting University Housing, the staff will notify housing staff, and *vice versa*, of the situation so that all parties are made aware of the situation and are in a position to proactively assist the student.

When students arrive on campus, it is their responsibility to make the residence hall staff aware of their allergy and to discuss how the hall staff should respond in the event of a reaction. Each student is different, so students are encouraged to have the conversation directly with their hall staff who would be the most likely first responders.

Students and parents need to remember to be as open and honest as possible during the early stages of planning their potential career at a university. The more information that is shared with the different departments early on in the process, the more the staff will be able to assist them and work to accommodate their needs before they arrive on campus. Early communication will also allow time for students and their families to sit down with each office and map out a plan for when the student arrives. Being able to meet and discuss how the university operates and what they can expect from housing and dining, helps to alleviate any concerns that the student and family may be experiencing as they make the big decision about which university will be the best fit.

> ***You Should Know***: **AllerTrainRA,** developed by Food Allergy Research and Education (FARE) and MenuTrinfo® is an online video training program designed for Resident Advisors (RAs) living in a dorm or residence hall on a college or university campus. The length of training is 10-15 minutes, and can be incorporated into existing RA training.

4. HEALTH SERVICES OFFICE

The Health Services Office should effectively generate, receive and process student health forms, provide health care services, including both management and emergency care, and coordinate health concerns with local medical facilities and providers. All staff should be trained in the health condition of food allergy, and how to recognize and treat an allergic reaction and anaphylaxis.

Best services should include:

- Providing training to emergency responders, including both professional and student responders, to recognize and treat anaphylaxis.

- Developing an emergency response plan that addresses how epinephrine will be accessed in a timely way, if needed, including on-campus emergency response vehicles.

- Where laws allow, maintaining a supply of stock epinephrine, and determining who may be trained to administer it.

- Providing food allergy education and anaphylaxis training to campus personnel, including student employees, in such areas as dining and residence life.

- Providing nutritional counseling with a registered dietitian.

- Providing counseling services with a licensed medical professional.

- Developing a coordinated program with the campus health clinic or city clinic/hospital.

- The campus health clinic should have a Procedures Manual that specifies how an anaphylactic reaction will be assessed and treated, how the student will be transported to a hospital setting, and who will be notified (student affairs office, the parents, for example)

***Insight*: Joanne Clinch, M.D., Clinical Director, Student Health Services, Wake Forest University**

Transitioning to college can be exciting yet challenging. New friends, new experiences, but for students with food allergies, finding a college that reduces barriers to eating and living safely can be an integral part of a successful transition. As a mother of a college student with food allergies, I am grateful to have been able to work with my institution and FARE to create guidelines for universities to help students live and dine more safely.

Student Health Services (SHS) on college campuses can and should play an integral role in assisting students in this transition. At Wake Forest we believe this assistance should begin prior to the student moving to campus. SHS asks all incoming students about food allergies or intolerances on their health information form. Students who disclose a food allergy or intolerance are connected with our campus nutritionist prior to arrival to discuss their individual needs and to answer any questions. SHS also encourages students to meet with one of our clinicians to discuss the ways our office can provide care and support. Support can include access to prescription medications, referrals to area specialists when needed, education regarding how to prevent exposure and how to access emergency treatment in the event of an allergic reaction. It is important to know prior to arriving on campus what services are and are not available for these needs.

Accidental exposures to an allergen can occur even when students are careful. It is essential that students know how to access treatment in the event of a reaction. Emergency response will differ from campus to campus. At Wake Forest University, our clinic is open 24 hours a day, 7 days a week. During this time there is at least one registered nurse on site who has been trained to recognize and treat allergic reactions. Nurses follow a standing order physician written protocol which allows them to treat anaphylaxis without a physician present, which can be life- saving. During the regular clinic hours SHS is staffed with several RNs and physicians who can monitor the patient, but after 5 PM our clinic staff is reduced to one RN. If a student presents with anaphylaxis after hours, emergency treatment is provided and 911 is called to transport the patient to our local emergency room where appropriate ongoing support and treatment is available.

Wake Forest is one of the few campuses in the country with 24/7 service, so it is crucial to inquire how care is provided on your campus in the event of an emergency. In some states EMS are allowed to carry and administer epinephrine, while other states do not authorize its use. If you plan to attend college in a state in which EMS cannot provide this treatment, it is crucial to ask if the university has a protocol which allows their staff to recognize and treat students using a supply of "stock epi" in the event of an anaphylactic reaction. It is also important to know the distance to the closest emergency room where full evaluation and support will be provided. Imagine attending a university where EMS and campus staff cannot provide epinephrine and the closest ER is 50 minutes away. Is that a risk worth taking? At Wake Forest we are fortunate to have on campus certified EMS responders who are trained and licensed to administer epinephrine and can be on the scene in under 5 minutes.

Emergency access to care is hopefully something none of you will require. Prevention is essential and college health centers can play a lead role in this effort, but it takes collaboration. One of the advantages of working collaboratively includes sharing of information and expertise that provides a holistic approach to supporting the needs of the students we serve. Student Health Service can provide education and guidance regarding the specifics of accommodations in the residence halls, dining services and classrooms. Disability Services can provide insight on legal obligations and best practices for the university. Our office works very closely with many departments to create a comprehensive approach to supporting students with food allergies. Integral members of the team are the students who live within the system. We often learn most from these students. One of the changes to our protocol came from meeting with two incoming freshman for a welcome visit. Each had asked for and received a single room accommodation for their food allergies. Both students would have preferred to have a roommate if they felt it would have been safe, but were hesitant to take the risk. I brought this information to our Housing Office who modified their housing application to ask students if they had a food allergy and if so, would they like to live with someone with the same allergy, if possible. Students sharing their experiences in the system help to improve the system. Gaps within the system can also be identified by engaging student involvement. While universities take measures to reduce accidental exposures to allergens, no system is perfect. At Wake Forest, when a student is treated for a reaction, our SHS meets with that student and connects them back to the campus nutritionist to investigate the gap so dining services can make adjustments to reduce potential future exposures.

Collaboration with campus partners and students can also help to increase awareness and reduce barriers to student engagement in and out of the dining facilities. Student Health Service can be instrumental in educating the campus and campus responders about food allergy prevention, recognition and emergency response. Paving the way to full campus engagement does not stop with campus staff. It is important that fellow students, particularly student leaders, have awareness of this issue and how to support their classmates. Wake Forest has worked with their "Invisible Disability" peer educators to achieve this goal. Physicians from SHS and the Office of Disability Services provided training to the peer educators about food allergies and Celiac disease during their annual training. Peer educators will move forward to educate their classmates, student organizations and RAs. This will promote awareness of how to recognize signs of an allergic reaction, how to support a friend with food allergies and how to plan events that include food to be safe and welcoming to students with allergies.

The number of individuals with life threatening food allergies continues to grow. Universities are exploring ways to provide safe options for living and dining. I would encourage students and parents to partner with their institutions to share insights and provide constructive ideas on how their college can address these needs. It is always so helpful to see an issue through the lens of those most impacted. Don't be afraid to be proactive and advocate for your needs.

FARE College Food Allergy Program

Food Allergy Research and Education (FARE) has taken a lead role in promoting the adoption of best practices necessary for effective food allergy management on college campuses by launching its *Pilot College Food Allergy Program* in January, 2014. This important resource, now available to colleges and universities across the nation, offers recommendations and guidance to help each institution establish policies and procedures that will allow it to provide a safer campus environment for its student population with food allergies and celiac disease. This significant effort will help advance a better knowledge and understanding of these health conditions as a disability, and establish universally accepted standards for their management at the post-secondary school level.

The twelve colleges and universities participating in the pilot program will incorporate recommended "best practices" for food allergy management into their policies and procedures in all areas of campus life. Modifications to this program will be made once the pilot phase has been completed and evaluated. The institutions participating in the FARE Pilot College Program are:

- College of the Holy Cross (Worcester, Massachusetts)
- George Mason University (Fairfax, Virginia)
- King's College (Wilkes-Barre, Pennsylvania)
- North Carolina State University (Raleigh, North Carolina)
- Texas A&M University (College Station, Texas)
- University of Arizona (Tucson, Arizona)
- University of Chicago (Chicago, Illinois)
- University of Michigan (Ann Arbor, Michigan)
- University of Northern Colorado (Greeley, Colorado)
- University of Southern California (Los Angeles, California)
- Valparaiso University (Valparaiso, Indiana)
- Wesleyan University (Middletown, Connecticut)

In June, 2016, FARE announced thirteen more colleges and universities have joined the FARE College Food Allergy Program. They are:

- Brown University (Providence, Rhode Island)
- Colgate University (Hamilton, New York)
- Michigan State University (East Lansing, Michigan)

- Purdue University (West Lafayette, Indiana)
- Skidmore College (Saratoga Springs, New York)
- Stanford University (Stanford, California)
- The University of Iowa (Iowa City, Iowa)
- University of Colorado, Colorado Springs (Colorado Springs, Colorado)
- University of Dayton (Dayton, Ohio)
- University of Illinois at Urbana-Champaign (Champaign, Illinois)
- University of New Hampshire (Durham, New Hampshire)
- University of St. Thomas (St. Paul, Minnesota)
- Worcester Polytechnic Institute (Worcester, Massachusetts)

FARE expects to have a total of forty schools signed onto this program by the end of the year 2016. If you are interested, you can visit FARE's website to see what schools are added over time to this growing list. Visiting the websites of the colleges and universities included in the FARE College Food Allergy Program will give you additional information about what kind of policies and procedures are in place to manage students' food allergies, on each of these campuses.

Insight: Kristi Grim, National Programs Manager, Food Allergy Research and Education (FARE)

College can be the perfect storm for students with food allergies. They're often living away from home for the first time, suddenly reliant on someone new to prepare every meal for them, and at an age when they are naturally prone to risk-taking behaviors such as not carrying their epinephrine or eating foods despite being unsure of the ingredients. At the same time, colleges and universities, although often eager to help, may not be equipped with the proper tools and knowledge to do so.

The positive news is that management of food allergies on college campuses is greatly improving. In 2014, FARE created the College Food Allergy Program to help unite students, parents, and colleges with the same goal: for students with food allergies to enjoy their college experience and to remain safe while doing so. Although each of these groups may have different ideas about how to accomplish this goal, when everyone works together and is properly equipped with education and resources, the college experience can be both enjoyable and safe.

The FARE College Food Allergy Program was developed with guidance from key stakeholders including parents, students, university representatives from a variety of departments, an advisor from the Association on Higher Education and Disability (AHEAD), and a liaison from the Department of Education. With this guidance, FARE created standard guidelines to better equip colleges and universities to support students with food allergies. Important components from the College Food Allergy Program include training opportunities for university staff, new student guides for potential and current college students, resources for student support groups, and the development of an online database where colleges and universities will share information about their food allergy accommodations with potential students.

Over the past few years, there has been a tremendous amount of positive change in the manner in which colleges and universities are accommodating food allergies, and many university representatives are extremely passionate about serving this community of students. But don't forget! It's also important for you to start preparing for college as soon as possible. If you haven't already, start learning to manage your own food allergies and advocate for yourself now. Make sure you're practicing those safe behaviors you'll need in college like: reading labels; disclosing your food allergies to food servers, friends, and dates; and carrying your epinephrine with you everywhere.

Education is key to staying safe with food allergies – in everyday life and on campus.

CONCLUSION

The majority of colleges and universities in the United States have some form of a food allergy management policy in place. There is, however, significant variability in what, and how it is offered, from one institution of higher education to the next. Safe practices to reduce allergen exposure on campus seem to be generally limited to dining services, with relatively minimal activity, at least in any organized manner, taking place in residence halls, for example.

We are on the horizon, though, for a positive change in the response of colleges and universities to the needs of their rapidly growing population of students with food allergies. There is a better awareness and understanding of this health issue than ever before. This is, in large part, due to the abundance of evidence-based information now available, advances in supportive federal and state legislation, comprehensive school management guidelines such as those developed by the Centers for Disease Control, self-advocacy efforts by students and families, and the vast work of professional organizations, such as FARE, who are committed to improving the lives of anyone affected by food allergy and celiac disease.

My message to you, as you plan for college, is to do your homework! Research the schools you are interested in to find out what is being made available so that you can be safe, have peace of mind, and enjoy all that being a college student has to offer!

TAKE AWAY NOTES

- ➢ The colleges you are interested in may differ dramatically in their response to the needs of their student population with food allergies or food restrictions.
- ➢ It will be up to you to investigate what is available to meet your needs, and what is not, at each school you have an interest in attending.

SUPPLEMENTAL MATERIALS

Studies Reveal Food Allergy Management Practices in College Dining Services

Perhaps the single most important source of information we have about food allergy management practices currently happening in college and university dining services comes from a research article published in the 2011 *Journal of Foodservice Management & Education*. This ambitious study investigated the views, practices and policies of dining directors who represented a total of 95 public and private colleges and universities, of varying size enrollments, across the United States. Each of these dining directors, who were all members of the National Association of College and University Food Services (NACUFS), answered questions on a web-based survey.

More than one-half of the directors who participated in this survey indicated that they are aware of allergic reactions, and even severe allergic reactions, happening on their campuses. Despite that admission, 54 of the 95 directors (56.8%) reported that there were no existing policies to address food allergens within their food service departments, although a relatively small number did express that they were in the process of formalizing such a policy. Most commonly, accommodations occurred only after the food-allergic students met with the dining service dietitian and explained their dietary restrictions and requirements.

How effectively were the needs of food-allergic students being met in these dining halls? The answer: based on theses 95 Dining Directors' answers to the survey, not particularly well. Although the dining directors were generally confident in *their* ability to identify the eight most common food allergens, there was a clear inconsistency in their opinions as to whether all of the full-time dining staff could do the same. Similarly, there was no strong agreement by the directors that graphics or icons were being used to indicate the presence of allergenic ingredients in foods being served, something that is obviously very helpful when we are trying to make safe food choices. The Directors also varied considerably in their answers about whether all dining hall staff had received training on how to properly administer an epinephrine auto-injector.

The good news is that this group of dining directors, collectively, seemed to agree that there is room for improvement. The majority of directors indicated that they consider the development of a training module for food allergy management as a very useful strategy for college and university dining services to adopt. In this way, they would be better able to provide a safe environment for their students with food allergies. More specifically, they identified food allergy training programs that grant certification upon successful completion of the training as being particularly helpful. This consensus was consistent, regardless of the size of the institution, its geographical location, or whether dining services were provided in-house, or with an outside food contractor.

Fast forward two years, when in 2013 the second study investigating foodservice operations at a university was published. Although there was only one university involved in this study (located in the Midwestern United States), the results provide us with some additional important and relevant information. Although the majority of food service employees who responded to the study's questionnaire indicated they were knowledgeable about food allergies, less than 50% could identify the eight major food allergens from a list provided to them. In general, these food service workers did not know that epinephrine is used to treat severe allergic reactions and anaphylaxis. Student employees, in general, had less knowledge and less favorable attitudes about food allergies, as compared with non-student employees. Of particular note: employees who received food safety certification, such as the ServSafe® program, had better attitudes about food allergies, and more food allergy training, than their counterparts who did not receive this certification. This finding strongly supports the opinions of the directors discussed in the previous study, who had expressed their belief that training which resulted in certification would be useful.

These important study results present compelling evidence that significant improvement is needed in the area of food allergy management in college and university dining services.

REFERENCES

Choi JH, Rajagopal L. "Food allergy knowledge, attitudes, practices, and training of foodservice workers at a university foodservice operation in the Midwestern United States." Elsevier, *Food Control* 2013; 31 (2): 474-481.

Rajagopal L, Strohbehn CH. "Views of College and University Directors on Food Allergen Policies and Practices in Higher Education Settings." *Journal of Foodservice Management and Education* 2011; 5 (1): 15-21.

CHAPTER TWO

Food Allergies And College Planning: Strategies And Recommendations For Students And Parents

"Plans are nothing. Planning is everything."
-Dwight Eisenhower

In the previous chapter we've reviewed the services offered by a college's **Housing/Residence Life Office, Dining Services Office, Health Services Office and Disability Services Office.** We've explored the variety and range of ways colleges and universities respond to the special needs of their student population with food allergies and celiac disease. Knowledge is power. Understanding how best to apply that knowledge is powerful.

In this chapter we're going to focus on these same four college offices with additional information to help you through the process of preparing for your college experience. I've provided recommendations for what can be done as you start this journey, for when you make campus visits, and also for when you are living on campus. Advance planning, as is always the case with food allergies, is an important key to success. With this approach, know that going off to college with a food allergy can be done . . . safely!"

These recommendations are meant to serve as a guide as you begin this journey. Use them in whatever way you believe they will help you most. The goal is for you to have made arrangements, in advance, to be able to safely eat and live confidently on campus . . . and get the most out of this experience.

A "WINNING" APPROACH

For the Parents

You have undoubtedly spent many years working tirelessly with your child's school personnel, particularly in the Pre-K through elementary grades, and have taken the lead in helping to insure procedures were in place to help reduce the risk of allergen exposure in the school environment. When your child was young, and you ate meals out at restaurants, you worked with the dining staff to assure that only allergen-safe foods would be served. You have carried your child's epinephrine auto-injector when he or she was at an age where you were always together. Know that you have been an important role model, and that your son or daughter has undoubtedly learned a lot about the importance of being knowledgeable, asking questions, planning ahead, and being prepared.

Gradually, you have been "passing the baton" as your child has aged and matured, and has been ready to take on more responsibilities. This transition is both important and necessary in order for your child to believe and trust in his or her own ability to stay safe. Continue to foster this independence. Your support and encouragement is what is needed most at this time for your child to develop problem-solving skills and the ability to self-advocate with regard to having a food allergy. You have all been preparing for this moment, so that your teenager feels confident and ready to handle whatever is encountered at college, and beyond.

The goal is to help make this transition to college as seamless as possible.

You can:

- ➢ Be available and offer support and advice when appropriate.
- ➢ Keep communications with your son or daughter open and positive.
- ➢ Assist in getting required paperwork completed and submitted to the college on time.

> ➤ Assist in finding a doctor located near campus, if needed, and help sort out any questions related to medical insurance requirements and Health

> ➤ Care Power of Attorney needs. Information about the role and responsibilities of a Health Care Power of Attorney can be found at www.americanbar.org.

> ➤ Demonstrate confidence in your son or daughter's ability to self-manage his or her food allergy.

Insight: **Anne Thompson, Parent of a college student with food allergies, Co-Founder, Mothers of Children Having Allergies (MOCHA)**

Preparing for the looming college launch is a process filled with hope and fear. Those are two of the more prevalent emotions I have experienced over the years. Hope that my child would be able to do anything that his heart desired and not be limited by his food allergy, and fear that he would accidentally be exposed to his allergen and have a reaction. Unlike sending him to kindergarten where I could make all the decisions for him, he now has his own (sometimes very strong) opinions about planning for his future that we don't always agree on. I have, for the most part, learned to pick my battles and sometimes have found it best to acquiesce and let him make his own choices even though I feel differently. After all, he is the one who has to "live it out" when I'm not around.

Going off to college is a very stressful endeavor for most kids. Having to manage one's food allergies at the same time adds a unique layer of complexity. Parents may question if their high school junior or senior is ready to navigate this terrain. Transitioning your child into the role of decision-maker should start early and progress gradually over time based on your child's age and maturity. Each step closer you get to passing on the "responsibility baton," means your child will be that much more prepared to make wise decisions when you are not around. Transition yourself into a coaching role well before high school graduation, and you will instill confidence and empowerment in your child before they leave the nest. I found that as I stepped back my son stepped up and assumed more of the responsibility for his safety. He became more empowered, and with that came confidence in his ability to manage situations because he was the one devising the plan. I feel very strongly that the time to pass the responsibility baton is while your child is under your roof so when mistakes are made you are around for safety and learning purposes. Parents must also model for their food-allergic child how to manage anxiety in numerous situations. Like it or not, our children read our emotions for cues on how they should react. If you are anxious, that will set a more anxious tone in the home, and your child will internalize this response. Have your young adult think through various scenarios that may arise such as: What will I do if new friends want to go to restaurants and coffee houses where it will be challenging for me to eat? How will I handle fraternity/sorority initiation or traveling with my sports team? What will I do if I have a reaction? Who will I train on how to give epi and recognize symptoms? Preparation and planning will help to reduce anxiety for both you and your child.

Remember too with reassurance that there are a great number of young adults who have already safely navigated their way through college and who have had a great time and gotten the education of their dreams. It requires you to research, plan and prepare well beyond the "regular" college search but it can be done. My son, in his early investigations into dorm life, chatted with several potential roommates on Facebook. After selecting one, the two agreed to share an allergen-free room. Many college food service departments are building online sites which include nutrition and allergen information for the food being served in their dining halls. Use these resources, as well as your on-site college visits during the high school years, to get a sense of how allergy-aware a college culture is.

My son recently had a reaction (his first after 3 ½ years at college). He called me the next day to let me know that he had self-injected, called the ambulance for transport to the hospital, and had a friend drive to the hospital so he had a ride home. I was so thrilled and relieved with the way he had managed the situation. His response was, you trained me well mom, and I did what you trained me to do. He has had years of training on how to manage his food allergies, and he proved himself capable.

You Should Know: In 2013, results of an online survey conducted by Harris Poll and commissioned by Mylan Specialty L.P., among 302 U.S. parents of children with severe and life-threatening allergies who participate in Valentine's Day activities where food is shared, found that:

■ Less than half of these parents (47%) talk with their child/teen/young adult with severe allergies about the potential risks from physical contact, such as kissing someone who has recently eaten their food allergen.

■ Among those parents of a teen who dates, only 47% talk with their teen about the importance of sharing the fact that they have a food allergy with their date, and

■ 35% of parents do not remind their teen to carry his/her epinephrine auto-injectors while on a date.

The survey results suggest that parents need to communicate openly with their children who have severe and life-threatening allergies early on when they are diagnosed, in an age-appropriate way. This approach needs to continue as children mature and face new challenges, including the potential risks associated with dating situations, such as kissing and physical intimacy.

Insight: **Linda Herbert, Ph.D., Psychologist, Division of Allergy & Immunology, Children's National Health System, Washington, DC**

During college preparation, it is normal to experience a variety of emotions. Parents may feel proud of their adolescent's accomplishments and excited about their journey into adulthood, but they may also feel worried about their child's ability to successfully transition into an independent young adult. The 'worry' emotion may be the predominant emotion for parents of adolescents with food allergy because they may worry about their adolescent safely managing their food allergies without parental oversight. Parents may question whether or not their adolescent has the knowledge, skills, and comfort level to be food allergy managers. However, it is important for parents to think about the transition of food allergy responsibility as a series of steps, rather than an 'all or none' situation. It's likely that you started preparing your child for independent food allergy management at college without even realizing it!

If you do have concerns about this transition and don't know if your adolescent is ready for independence, now is the time to start making a more strategic effort to help your adolescent take more responsibility. Think about the various tasks involved in your adolescent's food allergy care. Make a list of the things you do on daily basis (*e.g.*, read food labels), monthly basis (*e.g.*, check epinephrine auto-injector expiration dates), and yearly basis (*e.g.*, schedule an allergy appointment). Also identify what tasks you anticipate your adolescent will have to be responsible for while at college (*e.g.*, advocating for their food allergy needs in the dining hall). Then find the right time and place to talk to your adolescent about a transition plan. Together discuss what your adolescent can do now and make a step-by-step plan. Proactively provide opportunities for your adolescent to take the lead in food allergy management when outside the home. Continue to have oversight over your adolescent's food allergy management, but fade this over time. And remember to temper your expectations a bit, as adolescents will not do everything correctly the first time. It is also important to include your adolescent in medical appointments now. Although you know a lot about food allergy, it is likely that your adolescent could use a refresher. Ensure that your adolescent has time to talk with the physician privately as well, so that your child becomes accustomed to communicating with medical providers.

This transition can be stressful because you are comfortable managing your adolescent's food allergies and there is inherent uncertainty in letting your child take over food allergy management responsibility. However, by planning ahead and practicing independent care during high school, you are equipping your child with the skills needed for success at college.

For the College Student with a Food Allergy

I am certain that you have a tremendous amount of knowledge about what it means to have a food allergy, and that on a daily basis, you have been making decisions about what you need to do to safely manage it – especially in situations where you have been on your own. College will be an extension of these experiences. **Carpe Diem!** The future is yours!

This is an extraordinary time in your life; do all that you can to make it wonderful, rewarding, *and safe*.

First, some basic advice/reminders/responsibilities:

> Continue advocating for yourself by speaking up or asking questions when necessary when you are at your high school, or at a restaurant, and in social activities with your friends, for example. **You** have control over the questions you ask and the choices you make. If speaking up is something you are not totally comfortable with, and this is an area you feel you need to work on, high school is the time to practice whenever the opportunity presents itself. The more you take the lead with this, the more comfortable you will become with this role, and that will be important for you when you are a student living on a college campus.

> Make sure you know the signs and symptoms of an allergic reaction. Be aware that the symptoms may be different with each allergic reaction.

> Always carry your epinephrine auto-injector with you wherever you go, even if you don't think you'll be eating, and know how to administer it if you have a reaction. This is a mantra you have undoubtedly heard over and over, but if you haven't already done this, make it YOUR mantra.

> Learn how to cook and get comfortable reading ingredient labels, if this is something you are not already doing on a regular basis.

Doing these kinds of things will make the transition to college much more natural, when you are the primary person responsible for your own safety and wellbeing.

Insight: **Nancy Rotter, Ph.D., Pediatric Psychologist, and Lisa Stieb, RN, BSN, AE-C, Food Allergy Center, Massachusetts General Hospital, Boston, MA.**

Leaving home to attend college is both exciting and anxiety provoking for most college freshmen. The prospect of making this transition to college when you are a person with food allergies adds an additional challenge to this process. The importance of "readiness" applies to both general preparedness about leaving home, including being able to do things such as manage money and do laundry, and to specific issues related to independent food allergy management.

Most college-bound students will have had practice with label reading, ordering food in restaurants, carrying medication and communicating with friends about food allergies by the time they leave home. This experience will help prepare students apply these skills in new situations that arise at college. However, anticipating potential challenges and spending extra time in developing skills so that they come easily and naturally once you are living on a college campus, will be a good investment.

Practicing assertiveness skills related to food allergy management, prior to packing your bags for college, is essential. For example, challenging yourself by going to unfamiliar restaurants and asking to speak to the manager or chef about safe food preparation, even if you feel confident in the server, allows you to rehearse assertiveness skills. Repeated practice will increase your comfort with the process, which increases the likelihood of using these skills every time you need them. Some students find it helpful to role-play conversations about food safety needs with family and friends from home that are likely to come up in shared living spaces at college. For example, rehearsing brief scripts about keeping nuts or whatever you may be allergic to, off of shared surfaces or how to clean surfaces can be helpful. Additionally, practicing the use of a "matter-of-fact" delivery style for these requests improves direct communication.

While many teenagers have become accustomed to carrying their antihistamines and EpiPens® (or epinephrine generic auto injectors) without reminders from well-intentioned parents, this is an essential skill to master before moving out. Understandably, parents are anxious about the safety of their children, and sometimes both teenagers and parents get stuck in a routine in which parents ask if the teen has their medication (as well as other things including their wallet, driver's license, *etc.*) when leaving the house. Developing a step-wise plan to break such habits can be helpful. For example, as a first step, you can tell your parents that you have your medication before leaving the house, and if you forget, they can cue you by saying "do you have everything?" The goal will be to become completely independent in this skill well before leaving home.

Knowing how and when to self-administer your EpiPen® is important. This will help you to feel more confident when you are on campus. So that you are ready, make sure you are familiar with the signs and symptoms of a food allergy reaction. Know that when in doubt, it is better to err on the side of caution and administer your EpiPen® and call 911 immediately.

Getting comfortable with simple cooking and food preparation tasks is also very useful. Being able to put together something such as a salad or healthy snack container, so that you have back up food options for parties or events where the menu is unclear, can be helpful.

While college can certainly be a fun and exciting new experience, dealing with the stress of classes, meeting new people, living closely with roommates and the pressures that go along with college can be challenging. Having a plan for support from family and friends from home, as well as knowing where to seek support at college, such as the resident advisor or the college counseling center, can help prepare you for any rough spots you encounter, related or unrelated to food allergies.

PLANNING

IT'S ALL ABOUT FINDING THE BEST FIT – FOR ALL THE RIGHT REASONS!

The summer after sophomore year is a good time to begin planning. Junior year can be a particularly busy time: your academic studies tend to become more intense, you'll be taking the SATs and other standardized testing in preparation for college admission, and as an upperclassman, you may find yourself more involved in your extracurricular activities.

Going to the right college requires planning. Going to the right college with food allergies requires a little extra planning. Your focus will be primarily on the four campus offices we discussed in Chapter One: Dining, Housing, Health and Disability Services. Your actions with each of these offices will be different depending upon the phase of your planning. Make sure you allow the time you need so you don't feel rushed, and so that you can actually enjoy your search for the right college.

Here are my recommendations for your "Plan of Action":

PHASE ONE: GETTING STARTED – INITIAL PLANNING

STEP ONE: General Preferences

As you start to think about where you'd like to apply for college, my recommendation is to begin this process by figuring out if you have any general preferences that you believe would make a school a good fit for you. For example:

- Geographic location of the school
- Size of the school
- Academic strengths of the school
- Tuition cost
- Religious versus a secular institution
- Public versus a private college or university
- Four-year school versus a two-year or community school
- City school versus one located in suburbia
- Distance from home

***Make a list** of all of your preferences*. Then do a little research to find colleges and/or universities that fit with what you are looking for. You can do this by looking at college websites and by talking with your guidance counselor. Once you have completed your investigation, you are ready to <u>make a list of the colleges and universities that seem to match your preferences</u>. You can always add, or delete colleges to this list, as you plan.

TIP: It can be very helpful to have an idea how many institutions you are looking to have on your list: five, ten, more?

STEP TWO: Considerations Relative To Your Food Allergy

Once you have your working list of colleges, you can focus on these schools and begin to think about what you believe you will need in order to eat and live safely at college. Make a list of considerations relative to your food allergy that would be important for you to be most comfortable on campus. There are four areas at college to focus on as you do this:

> - Dining
> - Housing
> - Health
> - Disability Services

FOCUS AREA: DINING

What do you feel you will need in order to eat safely? Having dining service arrangements that meet your needs will be important. Some universities will have several dining halls located throughout the campus, which would give you the ability to choose where you'll eat, while other schools will only have one central dining hall. Some colleges will have a dining hall located in the residence hall for these students to take their meals. Many schools are now using computer software programs that have information about meals offered on campus, as well as information about food allergens and nutrition. Some dining halls will have ingredient lists posted by the foods being served in the dining hall, and some will have dedicated allergen-safe zones, which typically restricts gluten and some, or all, of the most common food allergens. Some colleges will train their food service staff in safe allergen practices, while others do not. More and more colleges have a registered dietitian available for you to work with to help you plan safe meal choices. At some institutions, it is possible to have a chef assigned to prepare allergen-safe meals for designated students.

***Make a list** of what you believe you will need in order to eat safely on campus.*

FOCUS AREA: HOUSING

Having housing accommodations available that you believe would be necessary for you to feel safe on campus, is also important. If possible, would you like the ability to choose your roommate? Do you think you'd feel most comfortable with a single room assignment, or would you like to have a roommate? Do you believe you will need an apartment that has a kitchen in order to cook your own meals? Although single rooms and apartment-style housing is usually reserved for upperclassmen, some colleges, based on your health diagnosis and related factors, will make exceptions to this to help find you a room assignment that best meets your needs. Some colleges have a kitchen facility in the residence hall that is shared space for all the students in the dorm, and you may feel that by using your own cookware, that could work for you. Many colleges allow you to have a small refrigerator and a microwave in your room, while at some schools, this may not be possible.

***Make a list** of what you believe you will need in order to live safely on campus.*

FOCUS AREA: HEALTH

Health services and emergency response services can vary significantly from one institution to another. Most colleges will have a health clinic on campus or within walking distance, while many universities will have a full-service hospital on-site. Some clinics are open twenty-four hours, seven days a week, and are staffed with nurses, nurse practitioners and physicians, while other facilities have more limited hours and staffing. Being at a college that has a pharmacy accessible by walking or public transportation may also be an important consideration for you.

Most colleges have trained emergency medical technicians (EMT) on campus, however, depending on the institution, these individuals may be medical professionals, campus police, or students. You should also be aware that not all emergency first responders are trained to recognize anaphylaxis and carry epinephrine in order to treat it.

***Make a list** of what you believe you will need in order to meet your health care needs.*

<u>FOCUS AREA</u>: DISABILITY SERVICES

The College Disability Services Office is the office on campus responsible to determine if a student's health diagnosis meets the legal definition of a disability. As we discussed in Chapter One, life-threatening food allergies and severe food restrictions generally meet this criteria. If you believe you will need formal arrangements made through the college or university in order for you to be able to eat and live safely at college, then you will need to work with the Disability Services Office. Reviewing the information on the website provided by the Disability Office for each of the colleges on your list will give you a general idea of how this office operates and the school's procedures for requesting formal accommodations. In your search, be aware that the name for this office may vary from college to college, and might also appear as the Disability Resource Center, the Accessibility Center, or something similar. We'll explore recommendations for your interactions with this office in greater detail in Phase Two.

<u>PHASE TWO</u>: GETTING PERSONAL – CAMPUS VISITS

Once you have your list of colleges that interest you, and your list of what you believe you'll need at college to live and eat safely, you will be ready to evaluate the institutions on your list to decide which school, or schools, are most likely to meet all of your needs and be the best fit for you. The best strategy to accomplish this: **campus visits**. There is, in my opinion, nothing more productive than making a campus visit to provide you with extremely valuable information about the schools that interest you most. Whenever possible, try and make this a priority. It is the only way to see what is going on, have the opportunity to speak with students who attend the college, and in general, "get a feel for it".

When you decide which schools you will visit, I highly recommend that you do the following:

STEP ONE: Official Information Session & Tour

Sign up for the **informational session** that every college Admissions Office will provide to prospective students. This is the college or university's opportunity to talk about features that can be found at their respective schools.

Sign up for an **official tour** of the campus with a student guide. This is also an activity provided by the Admissions Office. This is an excellent way to get a "lay of the land" and ask questions of your tour guide, who is usually very knowledgeable about the college. You can find dates and times when these informational sessions are being offered on each university's website.

Walking through some of the residence halls will give you the opportunity to speak with students who live in these residence halls, which can be very helpful. A Resident Advisor (RA), who is plugged in to what is happening in the residence hall and on campus, would be an excellent person to talk with, if you are able. Notices that may be posted in the common areas of the dorm and in the Student Union Center will give you a sense of activities and events happening on campus. The tour will also take you to the dining hall(s), and other places of interest, such as the Student Center, the Arts building and playing fields.

STEP TWO: Have a Conversation

Make arrangements for when you are on your campus visit to **meet with an administrator** from each of the four offices we've talked about: Dining, Housing, Health and Disability Services. This will be dedicated time for you and your family to ask any questions you may have and *have a conversation!*

FOCUS AREA: DISABILITY SERVICES OFFICE

If you decide to pursue formal accommodations for your safety at college, then the Disability Services Office should be your first stop. Make an appointment and have a conversation!

DISABILITY OFFICE – SUGGESTED QUESTIONS TO ASK

- Does your written Disability Services Policy include life-threatening allergies and related health disorders?

- What documentation do I need to provide of my diagnosis of food allergy or celiac disease, or other severe food restriction?

- Are the required forms posted online?

- Are the deadlines for all required paperwork also posted online?

- Will you coordinate my services with the other campus offices, such as Housing/Residence Life and Dining Services?

- If my needs cannot be met by college dining services, and there is a required meal plan, will I be released from this meal plan?

- Is it possible to be assigned housing usually reserved for upperclassmen, such as an apartment with a kitchen, if this is needed in order for me to eat safely?

- As a freshman, will I be able to bring a car to campus if I need it to be able to access groceries or health services?

- Who should I contact in this office if I have questions?

You Should Know: If staff working with you in the Disability Office doesn't seem very knowledgeable about the eligibility of life-threatening allergies for services, or what type of accommodations you may need, try not to feel as if this is a lost cause. They may simply need you to enlighten and educate them and bring them up to speed.

FOCUS AREA: DINING SERVICES

There may be a variety of dining options on campus, such as dining rooms located directly in the residence hall, larger community dining halls for all students to access, and even small retail food service areas or kiosks located throughout the campus.

You'll want to arrange a time to meet with a staff member directly involved and knowledgeable about the campus food service operation and have a conversation! This could be the Registered Dietitian (RD), the Head Chef, the Dining Hall Supervisor or Manager. You may find it most helpful to speak with a combination of these individuals. This is an excellent way to receive any guidance you may need to help determine how you will plan your meals and eat on campus.

DINING SERVICES – SUGGESTED QUESTIONS TO ASK

- Is the dining hall staff, including both professional and student employees, trained in food allergy awareness as it pertains to safe food preparation, such as how to avoid cross-contact, for example?

- Is the dining hall staff knowledgeable about ingredients in the foods being served, including the presence of allergens?

- Is the dining hall staff educated to recognize the symptoms of an allergic reaction and anaphylaxis?

- How are foods served in the dining hall? On a line by staff, cafeteria-style? Self-serve stations for students to use? Allergy-friendly food stations, which typically list the Top Eight allergens covered by the Food Allergen Labeling and Consumer Protection Act of 2004, (FALCPA), and/or gluten ingredient information?

- Can meals being served be pre-ordered?

- Are foods clearly labeled for ingredients and potential allergens in the dining halls? At food kiosks on campus? Are menus and ingredients posted online? Are ingredients in foods shared when requested? Do you have computer software apps that would enable me to access this information on my computer or iPad?

- Do you have dedicated areas in the kitchen for allergen-safe food preparation for staff to use? For students identified as having food restrictions to use?

- Is the Dining Services Manager always present in the dining hall when food is being served, should I ever have a question, or if I were to experience an allergic reaction?

- Will I be able to speak with the dining hall manager or the registered dietitian to help me plan my meals?

TIP: When you speak with dining services, ask them what resources they use to help students access ingredient information.

TIP: Make sure to visit the dining hall(s) at mealtime so you can witness exactly how it operates, and see first-hand what is being done for students with food-restricted diets, and whether or not a dining hall manager is present and visible.

FOCUS AREA: HOUSING/RESIDENCE LIFE

There will be similarities and differences in the residence halls and living arrangements at each college. There also may be differences in what the Office of Residence Life at each institution is willing to do in response to your having a food allergy. Arrange a meeting with the college housing office and have a conversation!

HOUSING OFFICE – SUGGESTED QUESTIONS TO ASK

- Do you provide students with documented life-threatening allergies or severe food restrictions housing arrangements that have kitchens, such as in apartment-style living, or in a residence hall that has a kitchen facility?

- Will I be able to have a small refrigerator and a microwave in my room?

- Would I be able to request a specific roommate?

- Does the college have a Resident Director (adult affiliated with the college, usually a professor or graduate student) assigned to live in each residence hall? Be aware that not all colleges do.

- Are Resident Advisors (RAs) trained in food allergy awareness, and/or how to recognize the signs of an allergic reaction and anaphylaxis? Are they instructed in emergency response procedures? Are they trained to administer an epinephrine auto-injector, such as the EpiPen®?

- Are safe foods coordinated with campus Dining Services for Freshman Orientation activities that include overnight stays?

- Is there off-campus housing available for freshmen?

- As a freshman, will I be able to bring a car to campus?

- Is there grocery shopping available on or near campus, and is transportation required in order to access these stores?

Author's Note:

Having worked as the Assistant Director of Residence Life, I know that staff in this office provides training to new and returning Resident Advisors and Resident Directors. RAs and RDs often arrive to campus before the general student population arrives, and will participate in programs to help them assume their responsibilities in this role. Topics covered will typically include learning how to connect with the other students and build relationships, developing skills in conflict resolution, recognizing signs of medical concerns, such as stress, depression, and substance abuse, and knowing important resources available on campus, for example. This is an excellent time for the Residence staff to receive information about food allergies, symptoms of an allergic reaction and anaphylaxis, treatment, and how to access emergency medical responders. *When speaking with the Residence Life Office, this is your opportunity to find out if they are providing education about food allergies to their RAs and RDs. If not, encourage them to do so!*

FOCUS AREA: HEALTH SERVICES

I encourage you to make an appointment with a staff member in the health service facility and have a conversation! By doing this, you will know the clinic's location and learn about the hours of operation. You can also learn what to expect if you need medical assistance, especially if that happens on the weekend, or in the middle of the night, for example. You will also be able to ask important questions to learn about the campus emergency response services.

You Should Know: Not all EMTs on a college campus are able to carry epinephrine, either because these individuals don't have the needed training and certification, or because the state in which the college or university is located does not have legislation to allow post-secondary institutions to stock undesignated epinephrine. As of the date of this book's publication, only three states allow stock epinephrine in institutions of higher education: *Indiana, New Hampshire* and *New Jersey*. Twenty-five states have pending legislation to allow for this, as well.

HEALTH SERVICES – SUGGESTED QUESTIONS TO ASK

Health Clinic Questions:

- Is there a 24-hour health clinic on campus? Is staff at the clinic equipped to handle a medical emergency?

- Is clinic staff trained specifically in recognizing and treating anaphylaxis? Are they trained to administer an epinephrine auto-injector? Do they carry these devices?

- Is the clinic staffed by registered nurses? Nurse Practitioners? Physicians?

- Is there a nutritionist or dietitian on staff in the clinic?

- Is there a psychologist on staff in the clinic?

Emergency Response Services Questions:

- Who is trained on campus as an Emergency Responder? Are they medical professionals employed by the university? College students who have EMT training? Are they EMTs employed by the local town or city?

- Are the EMTs able to carry and administer epinephrine?

- What is the average response time for a medical emergency on campus?

- How close is the nearest hospital? (This may impact response time to an emergency.)
- Where is the nearest pharmacy, and what are its hours of operation?

Timing

The best time to make these campus visits is during your junior year in high school, and the summer after, before you enter your senior year. If you are unable to make a campus visit, then make a phone call and have conversations where you can ask these suggested questions. This approach to planning is a practical way to narrow your list of schools and should enable you to develop an excellent list of a reasonable number of colleges and universities that meet all, or most, of your criteria in the categories most important to you.

Once you have completed all of your campus visits, you will be ready to make a decision about which colleges or universities you will submit an application. To sort this all out, I've included in the Supplemental Materials at the end of this chapter, a ***Master Checklist of Colleges' Responses to Food Allergies***, which you can fill out as you gather this information. As you review your notes, it can be extremely helpful to discuss your findings with your parents and guidance counselor.

When you have compiled your list of colleges that meet all, or most, of your criteria, submit your applications and look for the decision letters in the mail. These will usually arrive sometime during April of your senior year.

PHASE THREE: GETTING READY – AFTER YOUR ACCEPTANCE LETTERS

We're now ready to talk about planning after you've received your letter(s) of acceptance and have decided which school you will attend.

Here are my recommendations for your "Plan of Action" to help you get ready:

FOCUS AREA: COLLEGE DISABILITY OFFICE.

If you plan to request formal accommodations through the college, remember, it is your responsibility to make contact and initiate communications with this office, and not the other way around. You can meet with personnel in this office, or connect via telephone, to discuss and develop your health plan for required modifications to the school's programs and services you will need. Make sure that any requests for accommodations you are making are put in writing and addressed to your contact person in this office. Keep copies of all written communications with the Disability Office. You never know when a paper trail will become valuable to your efforts.

Although not always the case, be aware that if you are at least eighteen years old, it is possible that the institution will only want to speak with you about this process, due to legal considerations, and in its effort to maintain confidentiality regarding your health diagnosis.

Documentation. Most colleges and universities require you to fill out forms to document your request for accommodations or modifications to their program. Follow the instructions given to you, either as a result of discussions directly with Disability Office staff, and/or from information provided on the school's website.

You should be prepared to provide this office with a statement from your physician that identifies you as having a diagnosis of food allergy or celiac disease. If you have a food allergy, then the language included should indicate whether exposure to your allergen(s) could result in an anaphylactic, life threatening allergic reaction. Make sure you plan enough time to access any other information required by this office.

The wording and content of this letter is important. Although there isn't any prescribed language you are required to use, if your medical diagnosis meets the legal definition of disability, then this should be clear in the letter from your physician. You may also want to include additional information, which can be helpful as well, such as:

- Results of your allergy testing, although this is not always required, and
- Recommendations from your physician regarding special considerations you will need from the college's dining and housing services.

This type of information will assist the college in its evaluation of your case, its determination of whether accommodations will be necessary, and if so, the nature of the modifications it will need to make to the school's programs and services for you. Information you share with the Disability Office becomes a part of your educational record at the college. The ability for this office to share information in your educational record with other college departments, such as Housing/Residence Life and Dining Services, may be permitted under the Family Educational Rights and Privacy Act (FERPA) on a "need to know basis", in an effort to coordinate your services and accommodations.

Follow up with your contact person at the Disability Office if a reasonable amount of time has passed, and you haven't received a formal decision about what accommodations and modifications the school will make for you on campus. It is perfectly acceptable for you to request that they indicate a date by which time you should have a definitive answer. Again, do this in writing.

FOCUS AREA: DINING SERVICES OFFICE

Re-familiarize yourself with the dining service features of the college you will be attending. Begin to make definite plans about how you will approach eating safely in the dining hall, and work with the registered dietitian and dining services manager. If dining services offers an app with menu, ingredient and nutritional information, know how you will access this when you arrive on campus in the fall.

Consider getting a chef card to explain your food allergens to dining staff, and also for when you go out to eat at restaurants not affiliated with the college (FARE has a sample card for this purpose).

FOCUS AREA: HOUSING/RESIDENCE LIFE OFFICE

Once you have received your acceptance to a school, you will receive paperwork from the Housing Office that you will be asked to complete, and then submit back to this office. This form will likely include questions about how you would describe your personality and living habits, such as whether you are an early riser or like to sleep in, for example. The form should also ask for information about whether or not you have any preferences regarding your room assignment. *This is your opportunity to share important information about yourself and to request what you believe you will need.*

Food For Thought:

- Freshmen dorms: There are several factors you might want to consider as you weigh housing options available to you. For example, freshmen dorms may or may not have a kitchen facility to use, but they will be filled with students who, just like you, are new to the campus experience and are looking to make friends. Freshmen dorms typically also have Resident Advisors living in these residence halls who will be planning social events, especially at the beginning of the year. These opportunities to connect with other students will be significant in this setting and may be important to you.

- Apartment-style living: This type of arrangement will allow you to have a kitchen, which is clearly a valuable feature, but very often this type of arrangement has mostly upperclassmen who may have already established their group of friends. Apartments most likely won't have a Resident Advisor there to help facilitate social interactions. Very often, this type of housing is located further from the main campus, or even off-campus, where you might need access to public transportation or a car. You should be aware that most colleges don't allow freshmen to have a car without special permission.

It's important to think about the pros and cons of each type of living arrangement to help guide you in the requests you will ultimately decide to make and indicate on the housing form you submit to the college you'll be attending. Housing Office staff will review your information and make decisions about where you will be assigned for your on-campus living environment, and if you will be given a roommate or roommates, who they will be. You can expect notification of your housing assignment to arrive mid-summer, if you are scheduled to begin classes in the fall. *Once you have received contact information for your assigned roommate, it's a great idea to try and connect by phone, email, or in person, before arriving on campus for move-in day.*

You Should Know: Most colleges have programs to help familiarize accepted students with their campus, such as a Freshmen Orientation Weekend, which often include overnight stays. If you'd like to participate in one of these events, it would be a good idea to talk with staff in the Office of Residence Life, the Student Affairs Office, or the Disability Office to help make arrangements for you to have a safe experience.

FOCUS AREA: HEALTH SERVICES OFFICE

It's important for you to be aware that if you disclose information to the Health Services Office, such as having a food allergy, for example, this office cannot share this information with any other department on campus without your written permission, under the Health Insurance Portability and Accountability Act of 1996 (HIPAA). In addition to the services offered by the college's health clinic, you may decide that you'd like to have an allergist who has a practice within close proximity to your campus. This would be the time to investigate this possibility, and what limitations or restrictions, if any, might be involved with your current medical insurance. It's also a good idea to investigate the location of the nearest pharmacy where you can have your prescriptions filled.

Assemble a medical kit with all of your medications, including your EpiPen® and emergency treatment plan, and keep this in your room.

FARE has a form you can use for this purpose (see Supplemental Materials, Chapter Five).

Whether or not to wear some type of medical alert jewelry is, most likely, something you have already considered. If you currently wear a bracelet or necklace with this type of information, continue with this practice at college. If you do not, please reconsider, because it will provide your medical condition, such as your food allergy(s), if you have asthma, and whether you have any medication allergies, for example. This will be extremely valuable to first responders in a medical emergency, and will aid them tremendously in knowing how best to treat you.

Another consideration to discuss with your parents is whether a Health Care Power of Attorney should be in place for them. This means that they would be able to access your health information, and this would be particularly important if there is a medical emergency. If you are at least eighteen years old, this legal "permission" document is necessary. Be aware that some states require a specific form, and some states require that the signed document is notarized. An attorney will be able to guide you in this process, and you can find more information about this at www.americanbar.org.

As always, being knowledgeable and planning in advance will serve you well!

Insight: **Megan Yee, Northwestern University, Class of 2019**
Journalism Major
Allergies: peanuts, pine nuts

To be honest, I feel very lucky because my peanut and pine nut allergies have had very little impact on my transition to college. Northwestern University's dining staff is usually pretty thorough when it comes to listing allergens in the dining hall food, and the food provider tries to avoid cooking with peanuts in general. In addition, one of the dining halls has a separate station that serves food that is free of all the major allergens except fish. I steer clear of the desserts because baked goods tend to be risky regardless of who is serving them, but I can eat almost everything else. Northwestern's dietitian is also available to make personalized meal plans for students who feel unsafe eating the self-serve food at dining halls.

That said, I owe a lot to my parents for teaching me how to manage my allergies beginning when I was in preschool. They always stressed the importance of carrying an EpiPen® at all times, reading ingredient labels, and informing restaurant staff about my allergy. These safety practices quickly became habits, so I did not have to make any major changes when I started college. Having a solid handle on managing my dietary restrictions not only keeps me safe, but it also helps me feel like I have control over my allergies—not vice versa.

One suggestion that I have for incoming freshman is to get tested for food allergies before you leave for college, even if you think you already know which foods you need to avoid. I was diagnosed with a peanut allergy as a toddler, but I did not have another full food allergy test until my sophomore year of high school. I knew that kids occasionally grow out of food allergies, but I never considered that I could develop new ones. As it so happened, I tested positive for a pine nut allergy in addition to the peanut allergy. I'm glad I discovered the pine nut allergy through a supervised allergy test and not by having an allergic reaction after eating pesto in a dining hall.

TIPS FOR PLANNING

1.) **Timing** is an important factor. Allow yourself sufficient time to submit required forms and paperwork before move-in day. It is very likely that the university will have a prescribed timeline for this process; **make sure and pay attention to any deadlines that exist.**

2.) Decide if you will keep your current doctor, or if you will find a physician who is located on or near campus.

3.) Make an appointment with your doctor/allergist and ask for time enough to allow for a conversation where you can talk openly about going to college with a food allergy.

4.) Make sure to have all of your prescriptions filled **before** leaving for college.

5.) Bring your own dishes, cutlery and cooking pans, so that you will have what you need when you cook and eat. Do this even if you will be living in a dorm room as opposed to an apartment. If you can, buy distinctive items, or mark them in some way, so that people identify them with you and don't use them by mistake.

<u>PHASE FOUR</u>: ONCE YOU ARE LIVING AT COLLEGE

"Obstacles don't have to stop you. If you run into a wall, don't turn around and give up. Figure out how to climb it, go through it, or work around it"   *-Michael Jordan*

You will have many new and exciting experiences as a college student, both academically and socially. Living on your own will mean that this is the time for you to be your own best advocate, in many ways.

Important responsibilities for you as you manage your food allergy:

- Even if you have already met with the dining hall director and/or the registered dietitian when you were on your campus tour, I recommend that you check in with them again, once you are on campus. In this way, they will know who you are and can put a face to your name, which I think is important. You can finalize your plans and any arrangements in order to eat safely on campus.

- Carry two epinephrine auto-injectors with you at all times.

- Keep your emergency treatment plan with your epinephrine auto-injectors at all times. (FARE's Food Allergy and Anaphylaxis Emergency Care Plan is in Supplemental Materials, Chapter Five.)

> ***You Should Know***: In general, university personnel, such as college professors and dining services staff, rarely have access to stock epinephrine, which is another excellent reason for you to always have two of your prescribed epinephrine auto-injector devices on hand, at all times.

- Always read ingredient labels, whenever possible. Ask specific questions about the ingredients of a food you would like to eat, and NEVER eat or drink something if you are not 100% sure of the ingredients.

- Carry a chef card with you always that lists your food allergens and that you can use whenever you need to.

> ***You Should Know***: Use caution whenever you read advisory labeling on food products, such as "May Contain…", "Made on Shared Equipment with…", "Made in a Shared Facility with…"*etc.*, because the food may actually contain trace amounts of the allergen listed. A 2007 study which looked at the presence of peanuts and nuts found in products with advisory labeling, determined that 10% of these products did, in fact, contain traces of peanuts and nuts. This study also found that peanut protein may be present regardless of which type of advisory language is used.

- Share with your roommate and friends that you have a food allergy. Discuss with your roommate how the room will be kept allergen-safe for you.

- Share with your roommate and friends how to recognize the symptoms of an allergic reaction and how to use your epinephrine auto-injector correctly – they have "a need to know!" (One of my son's college friends called his EpiPen® his "Epic-Pen," a title which I think is awesome and very fitting!) Don't forget to let them know where you keep your medicine, both in your room and when you are out and about, and the need to contact emergency medical responders if it is used.

- Share with your Resident Advisor that you have a food allergy. Consider asking your RA if he or she would be willing to learn how to administer your epinephrine auto-injector. If conflicts related to your food allergy develop with your roommate or other students in your residence hall, ask your Resident Advisor for help. RAs typically receive training in conflict-resolution, and may be a valuable asset to you in the dorm.

- Think about how you will handle situations that involve food, both planned and unplanned, so that you will be ready. Read ingredient labels whenever possible, avoid food serving stations where cross-contact is likely to happen (think salad bars), and ask questions about food ingredients whenever there is doubt.

- Find and develop your support system at college. For example, develop friendships with people with similar interests who support you, or find other students who have similar health concerns, or utilize college administrators for assistance and guidance, when necessary. (There are some colleges and universities that already have a food allergy support group established on campus.)

- Ask questions and don't take risks when it comes to your food allergy – it isn't worth it! Keep it simple - if you are uncertain of the ingredients in a food or beverage, don't eat or drink it. Make good decisions so that you can reduce the potential for an allergic reaction and be able to participate, enjoy yourself *and* stay safe.

Insight: **Ethan Faust, Davidson College, Class of 2017**
English Major
Allergies: peanuts, tree nuts, dairy, eggs, barley, kiwi, sesame & shellfish

With so many life-threatening food allergies, I've been trained to be on high alert when I'm not eating what my mom has cooked. So going into college, I thought I would never be able to let my guard down and fully trust anyone with preparing my food.

The first week of orientation confirmed my fears. Every meal was pre-prepared and in a box on a table. There was no way I was going to believe that was safe. So I went 0-3 on meals my first two days, sticking to the Rice Cakes I brought with me as backup and dreading the next four years. I wish somebody had told me then what I know now. Orientation is not the norm, and it would get better quickly.

Once I moved to eating at the cafeteria after the conclusion of orientation, I was proactive about making direct contact with the people cooking my food. The first few days I would double and triple check with the chefs that everything was plain. But as I went back into the kitchen three times a day, I began to build personal relationships with the people cooking for me. In engaging with them, I helped develop a bond apart from the food. Through those conversations, I realized that the people cooking my food truly cared about my well-being. From there, I began to trust them. Slowly, the worries went away. But none of it would have happened had I not tried to reach out to the chefs.

Some people dislike the lack of variety that comes with the lone dining hall setup typical for a small college, but for somebody with food allergies, that system means only one set of people that I needed to trust. It allowed for the one-on-one relationship my allergies demanded.

Worrying about every meal is not sustainable for four years. Learning to trust was crucial. Orientation made me fear I never would be able to be comfortable. But once I developed relationships with the people who would prepare my food each day, I have put aside those fears. I still have to be cautious, but I have come to trust the people that cook for me every day. Once I was able to do that, I became infinitely more comfortable at college.

Insight: **Kathleen Shannon, North Carolina State University, Class of 2015**
Degrees: Human Biology, BS & Interdisciplinary Studies - Forensic Sciences, BS
Allergies: gluten, corn, tomatoes, apples, peanuts and dairy

I learned about my food allergies and intolerances the summer before my sophomore year at NC State. Since I didn't grow up with food allergies, I initially didn't really understand how complicated navigating a meal plan with food allergies could be - I just assumed I couldn't eat the obvious foods, like bread, pasta, *etc*. It was only when I kept having issues throughout the year that I realized I would have to watch out for hidden sources of allergens (especially corn and gluten). This really hit home a year later when I arrived on campus for my junior year and received a call from my doctor saying that my blood work showed an additional intolerance to dairy. I was distraught - I already had to be so careful, and throwing another restriction into the mix just added fuel to the fire. It was then that I decided to meet with the University Dining dietitian, to get some help. After our meeting, I diligently emailed her and her assistant every day to get full ingredient information on the daily menu items to determine, what, if anything, I could eat (something which I believe ultimately led to the availability of full ingredient information available on the Dining website menus). This continuous back and forth communication and deeper look at the dining options sparked an interest, so I ended up applying for a job in the dining program with the ultimate goal of helping to improve the allergy-friendly options on campus.

One of my favorite things to do in my free time was find new recipes and reviews on the many allergy-friendly blogs online, so the first food allergy project I started was the on-campus blog, "Allergy-Friendly at NC State." Every couple of weeks, I would review a particular dining location on campus as a "secret shopper" to assess their allergy-friendly options and cross-contact protocol, submit a report to my boss, and write a blog post about my experience. I absolutely loved this job because I felt like I was able to help other students find options the way some of my favorite bloggers helped me. A few months later, I expanded this role on my campus by joining a gluten-free brand's College Ambassador Program. As an ambassador, I started a student organization for students with food allergies - the NC State Food Allergy Support Group - through a partnership with the wonderful dietitians at the Student Health Center. The purpose of this club was to provide a community for those of us with allergies and intolerances, provide an opportunity to learn more about food allergies and related issues from local speakers in the field, and raise awareness for the necessity of allergy-friendly options on campus. This organization officially kicked off at the beginning of my senior year, and was a success. Like all new groups, we started out small, but the great thing about the group is that it represents an ever-present and growing group of students on campus, and therefore has the potential to grow into something impactful. Throughout the year, we heard from a great number of speakers, many of whom I met through my work as a blogger for gluten-free shows in my free time, and gained insight on a wide variety of topics. We learned about the physiological effects of allergens on the body, went to a gluten-free cooking Q&A with a local chef, and even toured a nearby gluten-free bakery! The most successful aspect of the club, though, was the fact that it brought a group of similar students together and gave us all a support system - something that is so important when it comes to health and adjusting to a new school.

My campus food allergy experience was an interesting one, since it started midway through my time at NC State. However, I think the big takeaways for me are the same as they would be for anyone attending college with food allergies: being informed and having an action plan. First of all, doing some research and educating yourself on the school's dining AND student health policies is extremely important. The more you know, the better equipped you will be to navigate the dining locations on campus. Many universities have extensive information on their websites, and I also suggest contacting the dietitian or dining manager at your school to set up a meeting. Figuring it all out on your own can be overwhelming, so it's nice to have someone give you advice! Second, don't be afraid to ask questions and continue learning throughout your time at the school. Sometimes, universities will have all allergen and ingredient information easily available to students. If not, asking employees or managers questions to help you figure out what you can and can't eat is definitely a good idea. Speak directly with an employee working in a dining location. If he or she can't help you, maybe they can direct you to a manager who can. Make sure you are paying attention to what you are eating as well, so that precautions are being taken from both sides of the counter. Third, be prepared! I always kept an arsenal of allergy-friendly snacks and staples, and medication in my dorm room and bag at all times. And finally, don't be afraid to get involved. My work with University Dining was so rewarding because I was able to help others like me manage their food allergy experience on campus. I encourage students to get involved and make that impact in their schools. Nobody understands food allergies better than those of us who have them, so we are a valuable resource when it comes to making an impact on campus food allergy policies and making a difference!

Insight: **Mackenzie Gannon, Ithaca College, Class of 2017**
Communications Major, Theatre Minor
Allergies: dairy, egg
Founder and President of the Food Allergy Awareness Club, Ithaca campus. Member, FARE

Transitioning into college is difficult for every teenager. Having a food allergy makes this transition even more daunting. If you are currently in college and have an allergy, you can most likely concur that we are the pioneers for food allergy awareness and education. Our generation started the buzz about this epidemic. Food allergies were basically unheard of until we came along. And now, colleges and universities are waking up to the importance of accommodating students with dietary restrictions. This way of life is not our choice, it's our way of survival. You must be your own advocate while at college.

For me, the worst part of applying to college was the application process. My thought was, why apply to a school that can't feed me? Therefore, I called every school I was planning to apply to and asked to speak to a dining hall representative, chef, school nutritionist, *etc*. The reactions I received varied from "Heck yes you'll be safe here!" to "What's a food allergy?" and then the occasional "No, we cannot accommodate you. Don't bother." When I received a positive response, I followed up with some emails and phone conversations, and eventually a personal meeting. It all came down to my gut feeling. If you don't feel safe eating, you're probably going to have a more stressful college experience. Food anxiety is sometimes unavoidable. But as a freshman, feeling comfortable and obtaining the right nutrition while away from home is crucial to success.

Although my school is very progressive when it comes to handling dietary needs, I saw there was room for improvement and growth. Therefore, I started the "Food Allergy Awareness Club". The purpose of the club is to advocate for those with specific dietary needs, serve as a support group, and create a safe and inclusive atmosphere in the dorms and dining halls. Students without dietary restrictions are also welcome! Our motto is: "Together We Can Find Solutions". I received wonderful support while starting this. Our advisor works in the marketing department for Dining Services and also has a food allergy. As a club we discuss improvements that could be made on campus, and then brainstorm with our advisor on how to tackle these issues. We've made great strides on campus already by reducing cross-contamination in food serving areas and increasing public awareness. I encourage all students with food allergies to become involved on campus in some capacity, whether it is through a nutrition club, student government, or starting your own club like I did!

The last subject I am going to talk about is something I am still learning to manage…something I wish I had an older mentor to help me with: "How do you handle food allergies in social situations while at college?" Personally, I find the biggest challenge to be explaining the seriousness of my allergies to others without scaring them away from being my friend. It's a sort of "darned if you do, darned if you don't" situation. I usually don't tell new friends about my allergies until we are in an eating situation. Even then, I'll order a "safe" food like fruit, or say I ate right before we went out, usually because I actually had a meal in anticipation that allergen-free food would not be available. Sometimes I'll just get a salad to push around my plate so everyone else doesn't feel guilty eating in front of me while I sit there. I never pressure them to choose a place where I can eat. One of the worst things is feeling as if you're a burden. If I'm going someplace new, I'll call ahead to alleviate the awkward situation of explaining my allergies while at the restaurant. My closest friend groups are always conscious about choosing a safe place. But with new friends, I like to go with the flow and not make a big fuss.

Unfortunately, I have not been invited to events because "I couldn't eat there" or "there was going to be pizza". I am sure many of you have experienced this as well. I then explain to these folks that unless pizza suddenly grows legs and learns to jump from their plate and into my mouth, I am fine with attending these gatherings! It's also fun to bring a favorite recipe or snack that I can eat and share. No one can tell that it doesn't contain dairy or egg! This seems to diffuse the situation.

Although I'd rather people be too cautious than careless, food allergies should never be a reason to be excluded. Nothing should be a reason to be left out!

As for parties and the like, NEVER GO ANYWHERE WITHOUT AN EPIPEN®. EVER. This is your excuse to buy a cute small purse, or simply put the EpiPen® in your pocket or coat jacket. Even if you don't think there will be food at the party, you should still have one…especially if you're going to be at all under the influence. It just puts your anxious mind at ease.

Which brings me to this point…if you happen to be kissing someone and you start to feel an allergic reaction coming on, perhaps you "suddenly have to go to the bathroom". I have had to run away from situations like that before. This is why you should always have medication with you, so you can take it immediately and take care of yourself and be safe. It's unfortunate that I've been embarrassed to tell the truth in the past. I've resorted to excuses such as "I felt sick and had to go home." But hey, that was not a total lie. If someone really cares about you, allergies will not be a point of tension in your relationship. It's important to be upfront and honest with a romantic partner so you feel completely comfortable. It will be a learning process, but someone truly worthy of your time will be happy to learn the ins and outs of food allergy safety.

I hope my insights have helped! College is a super fun and mind-opening experience, and I wish you all the best of luck. Never let your allergies hold you back, and remember to embrace opportunities to educate those around you!

__You Should Know__: A 2006 study published in the *Journal of Allergy and Immunology* investigated ways in which to reduce peanut protein in the saliva after peanut butter has been consumed. Researchers concluded that the majority of people who eat peanut butter will have no detectable peanut protein in their mouths if they subsequently 1.) eat a peanut-free meal and 2.) allow several hours to pass. They found this combination was actually more effective in reducing peanut protein in saliva than brushing teeth. *Doing this, as well, is still a very good idea!*

Insight: **Nicholas Ditzler, University of Michigan**
Chemical Engineering Major
Allergies: wheat, dairy, egg, corn, soy, peanuts, tree nuts, and shellfish
Founder, Student Food Allergy Network (SFAN), University of Michigan campus

When I arrived on the University of Michigan campus, I was surprised there was not a student organization for food allergic individuals to network and spread awareness of food allergies on campus. After seeing the need for such an organization, I founded the Student Food Allergy Network (SFAN).

One of the main goals I had when I started the Student Food Allergy Network was for the student organization to serve as a resource for kids that are at a transition stage in life. Whether you are transitioning from middle school to high school, or high school to college, food allergies can often make this process stressful. All our members have been in these shoes, and know just how difficult this process can be. By showing kids with food allergies that there are students who have gone away to college and are actively living with and managing their food allergies while still living a normal college life, we hope to relieve some of the anxiety and serve as role models for the kids who have food allergies.

There are many reasons why students join the Student Food Allergy Network. However, I would say that the single greatest reason is that SFAN provides a support network for those of us with food allergies. The Student Food Allergy Network is a great way for students to network with other kids on campus who also have food allergies. Many of our members enjoy sharing tips for how to travel with food allergies as well as recommending restaurants on campus that are able to accommodate for food allergies. The Student Food Allergy Network also serves as a great resource for students if they have any concerns regarding food allergies on campus. Many of our members know who to contact regarding specific concerns on campus and are able to help out.

One of the common questions we receive from high school seniors and college freshmen is how to find out if the University Dining Services can accommodate for their food allergies. One of the things I noticed when I was transitioning from high school to college was that the University was very accommodating and made sure I was set up with a chef who knew the severity of all my allergies. However, it does take some initiative on your part to make sure the University knows you have food allergies and need special accommodations. It is very important when you arrive on campus to contact dining services and see if they are able to accommodate your needs. I can personally say, after reaching out to dining services they have been very helpful and set me up with chefs who could make my meals properly without any of the foods I am allergic to. There are some students in our organization who did not contact anyone within the University about their food allergies and have had a difficult time making sure their needs are met. So I would recommend letting the University know of your allergies and need for special accommodations.

Going through college with food allergies can be stressful, so knowing some hints like this beforehand can make the process proceed smoothly. Like Chef told me, "If you don't tell me, I can't do anything about it. Actively communicating is the only way we can make this work." And a piece of advice: learn how to cook for yourselves, at an early age. This will serve you well as you transition to living on your own.

Social Aspects of College Life

The social scene at college is active and definitely fun, but you will want to have a plan for how to handle certain situations.

Alcohol

Alcohol consumption is a common occurrence at campus parties and social events. Please remember that drinking alcoholic beverages can impair a person's ability to make good, sound judgments, and when you have a food allergy, this may impair the ability to recognize symptoms of an allergic reaction. If this were to happen, it could make your response to this medical emergency slower than it would otherwise be. Muscles also become less coordinated with drinking, and that could impact the ability to administer an epinephrine auto-injector correctly, if it was needed. A slow and sluggish response to an allergic reaction is something that should be avoided at all costs. *Food Allergy Research and Education* (FARE) also points out in its **College Resources for Students**, that alcohol may increase the rate a food allergen is absorbed in the body. This is important to know because it means that symptoms of an allergic reaction may be accelerated.

You should also be aware that some alcoholic drinks may have ingredients that contain your food allergen. Beer, if it is made with wheat, should be avoided if you have a gluten allergy or celiac disease. Some alcoholic drinks have nut flavorings added, an obvious "no go" for anyone with a nut allergy. The same strategy you follow regarding foods you eat should be followed regarding alcohol – don't drink anything unless you know the ingredients of that beverage.

My message to you is be aware, think about this consideration in advance, and make good decisions! Don't share cups, or anything else, for that matter. If you put your cup down, and it is ever out of sight, throw it out. In other words, be smart!

Parties

Everybody needs time to relax and put work aside. For those of you who enjoy parties – there will be plenty! Some of these will be planned, and some will be spontaneous. Either way, it is likely that food will be present (and alcohol, too). For the parties that you know about, you can eat in advance so that if there is food present with unsafe ingredients for you, or you don't know what the ingredients are, you can take a pass and not go hungry. You can also bring food of your own to eat, as long as you take precautions to guard against cross-contact with other foods. For parties that are spur of the moment and food is brought out, if it contains your allergens, or you don't know the ingredients, keep it simple – don't eat it.

Dating

As you may have already experienced in high school, dating someone when you have a food allergy involves finding a way to communicate this fact, and sharing with this person that contact with your food allergen could result in a severe allergic reaction. It's important for you to talk openly about what needs to be done to help you from being exposed to your food allergen(s), such as avoiding eating any food containing your allergen, brushing his or her teeth, and hand washing. While this may be awkward, it definitely is worth it so that you can avoid any possibility of having an allergic reaction. This person will want to know, so that any risk can be avoided (which means having this discussion before the relationship becomes physical). If, on the other hand, your friend seems disinterested, or put off by this information, it's time to move on!

***Insight*: Dan Hanson, George Washington University, Class of 2013**
History Major, Sociology and Philosophy Minors
Allergies: peanuts, tree nuts

Having a food allergy is manageable. It can be a burden, a pain, frustrating. But it is manageable. The transition from High School to College is abrupt and exciting. Life changes quickly in a number of ways – but how you manage your food allergy should not be one of them.

For many of us, college is the first time that you live on your own, independent of parents and without the close supervision of teachers. You pick your own classes, buy or make your own food, and meet an entirely new group of people. You will face new challenges – but one thing remains constant: you need to be safe with your allergy.

I've had an allergy to peanuts and tree nuts since I was a toddler. When I was younger (when having a food allergy was much less common), my parents took care of me. They checked ingredients, spoke with chefs, made sure my classrooms were nut free. Eventually, as I got older and this responsibility fell on my shoulders, I had a strong understanding of how to effectively manage my allergy. I knew what steps and precautions I needed to take in order to be safe. I checked ingredients of the food I ate, spoke with waiters and chefs to make sure there was no cross-contamination, and told my roommates and girlfriends what they could do to help (in my case, this usually meant not eating peanuts or nuts around me). I managed my allergy in college the way I always had – by making sure that whatever I ate, or whatever environment I was in, was safe.

My advice to you: enjoy college. It's a tremendous time in your life. Whatever allergy you have will not define your college experience. Reflect on what you've done in the past to safely manage your allergy, use the tips and advice in this book, and apply those techniques to whatever new and interesting scenario presents itself.

If You Plan to Study Abroad

For many college students, going abroad to study is considered to be an important part of their college experience. It is an opportunity to live in and explore another culture, and that is an exciting proposition. This definitely can be done when you have a food allergy, as long as you include some important variables and considerations in your planning. The good news is that most students don't go abroad until their sophomore or junior year, which means you'll have many valuable experiences under your belt about how to live successfully away from home with a food allergy.

If you are fluent in a foreign language, then the country of that language's origin may be an option to investigate. It would be important to have a solid comfort level with your ability to communicate easily in this language to make the country a reasonable choice. If you are not proficient in a foreign language, then choosing a country where your native language is commonly used would be advisable. Either way, you will still be able to benefit from the experience of living in a foreign culture.

My recommendations for your planning, to help optimize your safety, would be to investigate:

> ➢ Paperwork the program requires; if it asks questions about medical conditions, ask what is done with this information once submitted.

> ➢ Whether there is a hospital in close proximity to the college or university that interests you.

> ➢ Whether the country(s) that interest you have epinephrine available in a hospital setting. If it isn't, consider choosing another country.

> ➢ Whether licensed medical professionals, such as doctors and nurses, will be readily available should you need assistance, either on the campus, or within a reasonable distance in the town or city.

> ➢ The types of living arrangements assigned to visiting foreign students. Would you have a roommate(s)? Will you have access to a kitchen (in which case you should make sure to have your own cooking pans and implements)?

> ➢ Legal requirements or guidelines that exist, if any, for ingredient labeling on food products. If there aren't any, this country may not be the best choice.

> ➢ Whether there is a main dining hall, and if you would be able to speak with the dining services director about safe food choices and menu planning.

> ➢ The food traditions that are practiced in the country you would like to study. These practices can vary widely from country to country, and some, such as sharing food or eating utensils, would not be advisable.

> ➢ Whether someone will be on the campus from the study abroad program, with whom you could speak if you ever had a question.

Whenever possible, speak directly with a representative of the study abroad program you are investigating, and have your list of questions ready. I also recommend that you speak with students (either at your school or from other colleges) who have participated in the program you are investigating, and find out as much information as you can about their experiences. If studying abroad becomes a reality for you, following these suggestions will help you to have a safe, and wonderful, experience.

Insight: **Tanner Elvidge, Northeastern University, Class of 2017**
Business Major
Allergies: peanuts

Studying abroad can be daunting, especially when you're heading to a part of the world you've never been to before. Not only do you have to worry about what to pack, but also about what food will be available in country.

I went to Cape Town, South Africa as part of a field study program at my university. It was an intensive program where almost everything was scheduled for us, including a lot of our lunches. The best approach to avoid any mishaps is to be upfront about your food allergies with whoever's responsible for planning the logistics – whether that's TA's or faculty advisors – well ahead of departure. Give them plenty of time to put in special requests at restaurants or with catering services and be willing to work with them as they're planning. This close collaboration will help ensure that any pre-ordered food will be safe and makes it much easier to work with your advisors in country if they order additional group meals. Plus, it has the added benefit of establishing a relationship with your advisors early, which makes the trip even more fun.

I was largely responsible for my own dinners while in South Africa as well. Luckily, English is the predominant language so reading food labels wasn't a challenge, but there was definitely some different food on the shelves. Take the same caution in foreign countries as you do at home: when in doubt, leave it out.

Conclusion

Knowledge + Support = Success

This has long been my mantra, and I recommend this approach to you wholeheartedly. You are beginning a new part of your life's journey, and being prepared and ready is, as always, extremely important. When you are planning for college, your parents and guidance counselor can offer you valuable help as you process your findings and make your evaluations.

When you are away at school, your family can continue to offer suggestions and advice when you need it. Your friends at college can be another wonderful and important source of support; it is a good feeling and reassuring to have people who "get it" and will "have your back." I encourage you to join **FARE's College Food Allergy Support Group on Facebook,** as another great resource for you. Consider starting your own food allergy support group on campus! Don't forget - college staff can also be an important resource for you when you have questions and need a little assistance.

Have confidence in yourself! Plan ahead, be smart with your decisions, and you'll be ready to fully enjoy this amazing time in your life!

TAKE AWAY NOTES

- ➢ Decide what preferences you are looking for in a college or university.

- ➢ Decide what features or accommodations you will need to help you manage your food allergy or food restriction at college.

- ➢ Make campus visits and make appointments with college administrators whenever possible to help you figure out if the college or university will be a "good fit" for you.

- ➢ Make arrangements for your safety *in advance* of your arrival to campus.

- ➢ Build a support network.

- ➢ Be aware of your responsibilities and make good decisions – in other words, plan for your safety on campus and don't take chances!

- ➢ The goal is to Be Safe and Fully Enjoy Your College Experience!

SUPPLEMENTAL MATERIALS

YOUR MASTER PLANNING "TO DO" CHECKLIST

√√√

INITIAL PLANNING

_____Determine general features about a college or university that interest you (size, geographic location, academic strengths, cost, *etc.*).

_____Make a list of the schools that fit your general criteria of interests.

_____Determine what features related to food allergy management are important for you to have at school.

_____Visit campuses of schools that interest you (when school is in session).

_____Attend Informational Sessions

_____Take Tour of Campus

_____Compile a list of colleges/universities that match both your general interests and food allergy considerations.

_____Complete all applications of schools you would like to attend.

_____Mail in all applications by the deadline indicated at each school.

AFTER RECEIVING LETTERS OF ACCEPTANCE

For Disability Services Office

_____ Make a list of any questions you have for the Disability Office.

_____ Contact the Disability Office, arrange a meeting and get the name of your contact person.

_____Receive (or download) all required paperwork from this office.

_____ Contact your physician and make arrangements for a letter to document your disability.

_____Receive physician letter of documentation of your disability.

_____Complete all Disability Office forms, with all required signatures.

_____ Mail all required Disability Office forms, including your physician's letter documenting your health diagnosis *by the deadline indicated* (Deadline Date is:_____).

****

For Housing/Residence Life Office

_____Receive paperwork/forms from the Housing/Residence Life Office.

_____ Make a list of any questions you have for the Housing/Residence Life Office.

_____Call or meet with Residence Life staff to discuss questions.

_____Complete all required Housing Office forms.

_____Mail in all required housing forms *by the deadline indicated* (Deadline Date is:_____).

_____Contact roommate(s) once this information has been given to you.

_____Tour assigned Residence Hall or apartment.

_____Make a list of all items you need for your college room, including dishes and cookware.

_____Purchase all items for your college room.

****

For Health Services Office

_____Receive paperwork/forms from the Health Services Office.

_____Meet with the Health Clinic Director.

_____Locate the nearest hospital.

_____Locate the nearest pharmacy.

_____Complete all Health Services Office forms.

_____Mail in all required health forms *by the required deadline* (Deadline Date is:_____).

_____Contact your physician and arrange for a prescription for at least two epinephrine auto-injectors and all other necessary medications.

_____ Fill prescriptions for all necessary medications.

_____Assemble medicine kit with two epinephrine auto-injectors, your Emergency Treatment Plan form, and all other required medicines.

_____Arrange for Medic Alert identification jewelry.

_____Make arrangements for a Health Care Power of Attorney.

****

For Dining Services Office

_____Receive any paperwork required by the Dining Services Office if you are requesting formal accommodations.

_____Meet with the Dining Services Manager.

_____Meet with Registered Dietitian and make arrangements for safe meals.

_____Complete all Dining Services forms.

_____Mail in all required Dining Services forms *by the required deadline* (Deadline Date is:_____).

COLLEGE COMPARISON CHECKLIST
RESPONSE TO FOOD ALLERGY

College/University Name	1	2	3	4	5	6	7
Housing / Residence Life							
Housing form has questions about health considerations including food allergies							
Housing form asks if special accomodations will be needed							
Housing has made accommodations related to food allergies in the past							
Single room or housing assignment with a kitchen is possible for incoming freshmen							
Resident Advisors/Directors educated about food allergies and emergency procedures							
Residence Life will coordinate with Student Services Office about Freshmen Orientation							
Health Services							
Student Health Clinic on Campus							
Pharmacy on, or near, campus							
Nutritionist on staff in clinic							
Psychologist on staff in clinic							
Will coordinate with the Housing Office to train RAs about food allergic reactions							
Trains campus emergency responders in anaphylaxis							
Campus EMTs carry epinephrine							
Coordinates with city clinic/ hospital							
Anaphylaxis procedures in place at Campus Health Clinic							

COLLEGE COMPARISON CHECKLIST
RESPONSE TO FOOD ALLERGY

College/University Name	1	2	3	4	5	6	7
Disability Office							
Clear information is posted on campus website							
Will meet with you to discuss disability services for food allergies							
Considers housing accommodations if requested							
Coordinates services with other campus offices							
Modifications/accommodations are put in writing							
Dining Services							
Director of Dining Services will meet with you							
Registered Dietician will meet with you							
Dining services staff are trained about food allergies							
Cooks and servers are trained in allergen-safe food preparation							
Dedicated equipment/surfaces used for allergen-safe food preparation							
Ingredient/nutrition signs placed next to foods served							
Ingredient/nutrition menus posted on college website							
Ability to pre-order meals							
Dedicated allergen-safe food stations in dining hall							
Ingredient information listed at retail food stores/kiosks							
Will assist with catered events							

CHAPTER THREE

What We Can Learn From Students With Food Allergies Who Have Experienced Life At College

"Tell me and I forget. Teach me and I remember.
Involve me and I learn."
-Benjamin Franklin

There are 17.5 million full and part-time college students in the United States, according to the American Academy of Asthma, Allergy and Immunology (AAAAI) in its fact sheet, "Off to College with Allergies and Asthma". Twenty-two percent (22%) of these college students have allergies. To put this in perspective, it is estimated that there may be 436,000-700,000 college-aged students with some type of a food allergy. My first message to you, if you are a high school student preparing to go to college and you also happen to have a food allergy, is that you are far from alone.

The transition from home to a college campus is considerable. While this move is, in many ways, exciting, it can also present new challenges. It is a pretty sure bet that as a college freshman, you will be exposed to different people, different ideas, and different activities than you've previously experienced. You will be making decisions about a broad range of things, including everything from academic course work to social situations. If you are like most college freshmen, this may be the first time you will find yourself living independently. In this new role you will be the person "in charge" and responsible for everyday life, including managing your food allergy. All of this may be something you are looking forward to, but also be a little nervous about, as well. My message to you, again, is that if any of this describes you, you are not alone.

Food allergy attitudes among young adults and college students

Although there is not a tremendous amount of information available to us which explores the attitudes and behaviors of college-aged students living with a food allergy, there have been a handful of research studies which were designed to address this subject. These studies provide us with important findings and help us to have a better understanding of what the combination of having a food allergy and being a college student may mean. In this chapter, you will read about the different ways these students approached and handled a variety of situations they encountered on campus, as it related to their food allergy. My hope is that this will be helpful and informative for you as a prospective student planning for college, because you will likely face similar scenarios.

The information covered in this chapter will give an overview of the many ways having a food allergy may impact the college experience for a student with this diagnosis. Understanding the challenges involved and this potential impact should make clear why a college's approach to food allergy management should be an important consideration.

Here's what we know:

A significant number of the students in these studies revealed engaging in "risk-taking" behaviors in the management of their food allergy. Findings from a 2009 study conducted on the University of Michigan, Ann Arbor campus, indicate that approximately 40% of students responding to an online survey reported *always* avoiding foods to which they are allergic.

Another study investigating the behaviors of adolescents and young adults found that some of these individuals intentionally ingested a known food allergen. In fact, based on the results of this internet-based, anonymous questionnaire, 54% of the students who answered said they had, at one time or another, purposefully eaten a potentially allergenic food.

Another risk-taking trend seen from research results is the decision not to carry a prescribed epinephrine auto-injector device. Of the 287 undergraduates in the University of Michigan study who reported having a food allergy, only 21%, indicated that they made arrangements to maintain their epinephrine, and even less, 6.6%, said they *always* carry this life-saving device. Students who had a peanut or tree nut allergy were more likely to always carry their self-injectable epinephrine as compared with students who had other food allergies, although no insights or reasons for this were discussed in the study.

A particularly disturbing finding in the Michigan study was the fact that 27.7% of these students reported never having been prescribed an epinephrine auto-injector by their physician, despite having been diagnosed with a food allergy. Not carrying an epinephrine device, either by personal decision, or because it wasn't prescribed, is clearly problematic. Not having immediate access to epinephrine to treat a severe allergic reaction will result in some kind of a delay in administering this life-saving medicine: this is considered a risk factor for fatal anaphylaxis. Information revealed in these studies did not indicate why epinephrine had not been prescribed in these cases, or if the students with a food allergy who had not been given a prescription for an epinephrine auto-injector were aware of its critical role in treating anaphylaxis.

We know from these studies that there is evidence that allergic reactions are happening on college campuses. A long-term study conducted from 1994 to 2004 found that out of 63 food-allergic reactions that resulted in fatalities, 16 involved college-aged students, and 50% of the reactions occurred on college campuses. In the University of Michigan study, 57% of the students said they had experienced an allergic reaction to food, and of these incidents, 36.2% of the symptoms they reported were consistent with anaphylaxis. It appears that these allergic reactions happened in a variety of locations on campus. For example, approximately 62% of the students in this study reported having experienced an allergic reaction in either their residence hall or the dining hall.

Many of these students expressed having concerns about practices they encountered in their campus dining halls that did not allow them to eat safely. For example, they reported that foods served were not always labeled with ingredients and listed allergens. One-third of these students (32.7%) reported being worried about being exposed to allergenic foods in their dining hall.

The decision to communicate information about having a food allergy to others was not a common practice among many of the college students who participated in these studies. When this was shared, it was entrusted most often to a close housemate or roommate. These conversations, however, did not typically also include how to recognize the symptoms of an allergic reaction, or how to treat one. A significant number of these college students indicated that they were much less likely to share their diagnosis with health services on campus. Campus dining service personnel, it turns out, were the least likely to be notified of any diet or food restrictions.

These research studies offered possible explanations for some of the risky behaviors described on campus. Most significantly, they suggest that for some of these young adults, assuming the primary role and responsibility for managing their food allergies may have been something which these college students were not yet comfortable. In other words, decisions that resulted in putting them at risk for allergen exposure may be a reflection of their making adjustments to a role they may not have had before arriving on campus. For other students, they speculate that reckless decision-making may have been influenced by the desire to not appear differently, in any significant way, from their peers.

I would like to add my perspective regarding possible explanations for some of the decisions made by the students in these studies. First, the lack of notification by these students to campus health and dining services about having a food allergy may be a reflection of the fact that many colleges and universities do not have protocols and procedures in place to facilitate the receipt, or processing, of this kind of information. It is plausible that some of these students may not have had a format by which to provide this information. In addition, students with food allergies have to handle attitudes, both supportive and negative, from individuals within their college community. We all know, and have experienced, occasions where certain people have been uninformed, insensitive, or even unkind, when the topic of food allergy is discussed. Perhaps in response to this reality, in part, it is possible that some students who participated in these studies chose not to be forthcoming in sharing information about their food allergy with either college personnel or their peers.

Suggestions Made by College Students Living with a Food Allergy

Students participating in these studies have revealed important information about what they believe would improve their ability to manage their food allergies more easily at college. They stated they would find helpful:

➢ A more supportive college environment.

➢ To receive information about food allergy accommodations during campus orientation.

➢ Food allergy education to be provided for the other students.

➢ Staff members identified to them who they could speak with about meals.

➢ A wider selection of allergen-free meal options.

> ➢ Having food allergy labels on foods being served that are easy to read.

Conclusion

The challenges to stay safe on a college or university campus can be, at times, overwhelming. The trends in attitudes, behaviors, and experiences of college students with a food allergy help us to understand that there are many factors that can affect how college students manage their food allergies. Some undergraduates appear to carry their prescribed epinephrine, avoid allergenic foods and share with their friends the fact that they have a food allergy. Others are not as consistent in doing these things, and as a result, put themselves at risk for allergen exposure and experiencing an allergic reaction. All of the students who answered these surveys, and chose to reveal personal information, deserve a tremendous amount of credit, and our thanks. We can learn a lot from their answers and their experiences.

TAKE AWAY NOTES

> ➢ This is likely the first time that most college students with a food allergy will be living on their own.

> ➢ This transition will present new challenges and experiences when these students are primarily responsible for their safety and well-being.

> ➢ Risk-taking behaviors which include eating foods which may contain allergens, not carrying prescribed epinephrine auto-injectors, and not informing friends or campus authorities, such as dining services, about having a food allergy and other related health needs, may contribute to the potential for having an allergic reaction and anaphylaxis.

> ➢ To help reduce the risk of a severe allergic reaction, it is important to understand the potential risks for allergen exposure in the college environment, to have a plan to avoid these risks whenever possible, and to be prepared to respond should anaphylaxis occur.

> ➢ College students would like to see improved practices by college staff and the administration to allow them to manage their food allergies more easily.

CHAPTER FOUR

Understanding The Laws That Protect
College Students With Food Allergies

*"A law is valuable not because it is a law, but
because there is right in it."*
-Henry Ward Beecher

There are state and federal laws and regulations which have been constructed to protect the rights and privileges of individuals with disabilities, and that includes students with documented life-threatening food allergies. The federal civil rights laws which are most often referred to when we speak about students with life-threatening food allergies are *Section 504 of the Rehabilitation Act of 1973* (**Section 504**), and the *Americans with Disabilities Act of 1990* (**ADA**). The discussion of the laws covered in this chapter will help to:

1. Clarify their meaning, and

2. Highlight how they apply to institutions of higher education and impact their obligation to respond to the needs of students identified to them as having a food allergy.

"Allergy" Defined as a Disability

Although general confusion over whether a student with a life-threatening food allergy is considered to have a disability under the law is beginning to dissipate, a brief review of this issue may be helpful. Under the ADA and Section 504, a disability is defined as a physical or mental impairment that substantially limits one or more major life activities. A physical or mental impairment is defined as "any physiological disorder or condition . . . affecting one or more body systems." A "major life activity" would include such things as seeing, hearing, breathing, eating and learning. We know that an individual with a food allergy may experience substantially limited breathing during anaphylaxis due to the involvement of the body's respiratory system. The physiological condition of a food allergy may also affect the digestive, skin and cardiovascular body systems. Bottom line - a life-threatening food allergy generally meets the criteria of a qualifying impairment, and as such, meets the definition of a disability.

The Office for Civil Rights (OCR), within the United States Department of Education, recognizes *allergy* as a "hidden disability," which it defines as "physical or mental impairments that are not readily apparent to others." This is important to understand when you engage in discussions with college administration, particularly if there are questions asked about the appropriateness of accommodations for a college student with food allergies. More information about the specific language used to define a qualified individual with a disability can be found by searching 28 C.F.R. § 35.104.

The Americans With Disabilities Act of 1990 (ADA)

The Americans with Disabilities Act of 1990, most often referred to as the ADA, is a federal civil rights law. It was constructed with the clear purpose of eliminating discrimination against anyone with a disability. Its language provides mandates which are intended to set standards to insure that people with disabilities have opportunities equal to people without disabilities. The law clearly states that " . . . no individual shall be discriminated against on the basis of disability in the full and equal enjoyment of the goods, services, facilities, privileges, advantages . . . of any place of public accommodation . . ." The ADA requires that colleges and universities have policies in place that serve to guide the process for the institution to meet the special needs requested by the student with a disability.

The ADA is administered by the Department of Justice (DOJ).

ADA, Title II and Title III

There are two sections called "Titles" within the ADA which may be applied to students with life-threatening food allergies:

Title II: The requirements of Title II are similar to the requirements found in Section 504. It states that qualified persons with a disability may not be ". . .excluded from participation in or be denied the benefits of services, programs or activities of a public entity. . ." A "public entity" may be defined as any state or local government or its agency. A public school, such as a state college or university, is an example of a government agency. Title II, therefore, protects individuals with disabilities in state and local government agencies and programs and requires these programs to be readily accessible to them. The implementing regulation for Title II can be found at 28 C.F.R. Part 55.

Public institutions of higher education, under the ADA, must provide *reasonable* accommodations that would allow their disabled students to participate safely and have equal opportunity to benefit in programs offered by the school. What is considered "reasonable?" Under the ADA, a public college is not required to provide an accommodation if it can prove that it would result in an "undue burden", such as necessitating a fundamental change to its program or create excess and undue financial burden to that institution.

Title III: Title III of the ADA extends these same rights to individuals with disabilities in places of public accommodation *regardless of whether they receive federal funds*. This makes the requirements presented by the ADA broader than those found under Section 504. The definition of places of public accommodation by a *private* entity include: "a nursery, elementary, secondary, *undergraduate or postgraduate private school*." In other words, college students with diagnosed life-threatening food allergies who attend a private college or university are entitled to the same benefits of their education as their nondisabled classmates. Like their public counterparts, these private institutions must be prepared to appropriately handle the needs of their students with a medical diagnosis of food allergy and provide reasonable accommodations.

The only institutions of higher education that are exempt from the requirements of the ADA are colleges or universities that are 1.) operated by a religious organization, and 2.) do not receive any type of federal funding. The small number of schools in the United States that fit this description do not have any legal obligation to provide accommodations to their students with disabilities. A religious college that *does* receive any form of federal monies, however, is subject to the requirements of Section 504 of the Rehabilitation Act.

The ADA Amendments Act of 2008 (ADAAA, 2008), which went into effect on January 1, 2009, broadened the scope of the interpretation of the definition of disability. The major changes made by these amendments were:

    1.) Expanding major life activities to include such things as eating and bodily functions,

2.) No longer requiring medical supplies or prosthetics as criteria used to determine   substantial limitation of a major life activity,

3.) Adding conditions that are episodic, and

4.) Determining that the definition of disability under Section 504 and the ADA be "in favor of broad coverage…to the maximum extent permitted by [its] terms"
42 U.S.C. (§ 12102[4][A]).

Section 504 of the Rehabilitation Act of 1973 (PL 93-112)

Section 504 is a federal civil rights law constructed to protect the rights of individuals with a disability and is meant to: "prohibit discrimination on the basis of disability in education . . . in any program or institution receiving federal funds". Students who have a medical diagnosis of a life-threatening allergy are generally considered to have a disability, and are likely eligible for protection under Section 504 of the Rehabilitation Act of 1973.

Section 504 is administered by the Office for Civil Rights (OCR), within the U.S. Department of Education.

What this means is that any public educational institution or program that receives federal funding, for any reason, must comply with the requirements found under Section 504. Colleges, both two-year and four-year, and universities that receive some type of financial assistance from the U.S. Department of Education, must be in compliance with Section 504. For institutions that receive federal money, they are, in effect, agreeing to a contract with the government which says they agree not to discriminate against anyone with a disability and they will uphold the requirements set forth in this law. You will find that most, if not all, public colleges and universities, receive some form of federal funding. Private schools are also required to comply with the provisions found under Section 504 if they receive federal funding for any reason, as well. The regulations that implement Section 504, as it pertains to educational institutions, can be found at: 34 C.F.R. Part 104.

For college students with a food allergy that meets the legal definition of disability, the implications of this law are important to understand. Although a college or university is not required to ensure that students identified to them as having a disability receive a Free Appropriate Education (often referred to as FAPE), which is the legal requirement for Kindergarten through grade twelve, it must provide reasonable modifications to the school's policies, programs, practices and procedures, so that these students have equal access and the ability to benefit from the programs being offered. These accommodations may mean that adjustments are made to the academic, housing or dining programs, when necessary. For example, in order to accommodate a student with a food allergy or celiac disease, the college housing office may provide a room assignment that allows the student to access kitchen facilities, either in the room, or in the residence hall. Similarly, the institution's dining services may offer the means for the student to access allergen-free foods on campus.

Family Educational Rights and Privacy Act (FERPA)

The purpose of FERPA, a federal law, is to protect the privacy of student's "education records". Education records are records that directly relate to a specific student and are maintained by an educational agency or institution. FERPA applies to all educational agencies and institutions that receive funding under any program administered by the U.S. Department of Education. Under FERPA, in an educational setting, information about a student's health becomes a part of the student's education record and may be shared with appropriate school officials when such knowledge is essential to protect the health and well-being of the student. These school officials are considered to have a legitimate "need to know' in order to help them protect the welfare of the student.

For more information about FERPA, contact: Family Policy Compliance Office, U.S. Department of Education, 400 Maryland Avenue, S.W., Washington, D.C. 20202-8520, or go to: www.ed.gov/policy/gen/guid/fpco/index.html.

Health Insurance Portability and Accountability Act of 1996 (HIPAA)

HIPAA established national standards for electronic health care transactions to protect the privacy of an individual's health information. Health care providers, including institutions such as hospitals and health clinics, as well as individual physicians and practitioners, are entities subject to the requirements of HIPAA. The HIPAA Privacy Rule requires health care providers to have safeguards in place to protect a patient's privacy, including setting appropriate limits related to the use and disclosure of a patient's information without authorization.

For more information about HIPAA, go to: www.hhs.gov/ocr/hipaa.

To understand the application of FERPA and HIPAA to student health records, go to: www2.ed.gov/policy/gen/guid/fpco/doc/ferpa-hipaa-guidance.pdf.

You Should Know: **Legal Requirements for Institutions of Higher Education:**

1.) Under the ADA and Section 504, there is no "Child Find" obligation to identify students with disabilities imposed upon institutions of higher education, despite the fact that this is a legal requirement that exists for grades K-12. What does this mean for you? You, as the student, are responsible for providing written documentation of your disability to the college or university's Disability Office. Examples of documentation include the results from medical or psychological tests administered by your physician or other professional, for example.

2.) A qualified student with a disability at the postsecondary level must meet the academic standards required for admission to the college.

3.) Under Section 504, a college or university may not inquire, prior to your admission, about whether or not you, as an applicant, have a disability.

4.) Under Section 504, the college or university must inform you of services available, and the name of the person at the institution who is responsible for implementing the requirements of Section 504.

5.) The law requires that accommodations made by the college for a disabled student must be approved in writing.

6.) The postsecondary institution must have a grievance procedure if you believe your special needs are not being adequately met. The person to contact would be the staff member in the school's Disability Services Office who has the responsibility to coordinate its compliance with Section 504 and Title II or Title III of the ADA.

Lesley University Settlement (DJ 202-36-231)

Several years ago, a landmark case occurred involving several college students with celiac disease and Lesley University, a private, four-year, nonprofit university located in Cambridge, Massachusetts. This was the first food allergy-related settlement under the ADA in higher education, and it has significant implications for college students with celiac disease and food allergies.

Nature of complaint

The students involved filed a formal complaint with the United States Department of Justice (DOJ) in October, 2009, stating Lesley University was not making the necessary accommodations for them to be able to safely eat food prepared by dining services on campus, which was a violation of Title III of the Americans with Disabilities Act of 1990 (42 U.S.C. §§ 12181-12189). Title III prohibits a private university from discriminatory activities against an individual on the basis of disability, in the full and equal enjoyment of the university's services, facilities, privileges, or accommodations, for example. In a related fact, Lesley University required these students to purchase the meal plan offered by the school, despite their inability to safely consume school-prepared foods.

Outcome

After an investigation, the DOJ found that Lesley University had violated Title III of the ADA, and had failed to make the necessary and reasonable accommodations in its "policies, practices and procedures to permit students with celiac disease and/or food allergies…to fully and equally enjoy the privileges, advantages, and accommodations of its food service and meal plan system." (DOJ, *Settlement Agreement between the United States of America and Lesley University*. DJ 202-36-231.)

Significantly, the judgment found that food allergies may constitute a disability under the ADA.

Nature of agreement/resolution

As a result of the settlement, Lesley University agreed to provide and implement practices that are in compliance with the ADA, so that students with food allergies and celiac disease would be ensured full and equal enjoyment of the University's meal plan and dining services. The press release issued by the Office of Public Affairs for the U.S. Department of Justice cited many of the terms of the settlement, including that the University must:

- Provide gluten-free and allergen-free food options in its dining hall food lines,
- Post signs identifying specific food allergens and gluten in all of its five cafeterias,
- Allow students identified to them as having a food allergy, to pre-order allergen-free meals,
- Provide dedicated space in the college's kitchens to store and prepare gluten-free and allergen-free food, to accommodate students concerned about cross-contact,
- Provide training to food service and University staff about food allergy-related issues,
- Endeavor to retain vendors that accept students' prepaid meal cards and also offer food free of allergens,
- Allow students to be exempt from the mandatory meal plan,
- Ensure that the University's Disability Services Office works with each student who is identified to them as having a food allergy or celiac disease, and develop a written, individualized modification plan, and
- Pay $50,000 in compensatory damages to the students who have celiac disease or other food allergies who filed the complaint.

The DOJ's press release included the following message: "By implementing this agreement, Lesley University will ensure students with celiac disease and other food allergies can obtain safe and nutritional food options" said Thomas E. Perez, Assistant Attorney General for the Civil Rights Division. "This agreement ensures that Lesley's meal program is attentive to the schedules and demands of college students with food allergies, an issue colleges and universities across the country need to consider."

The settlement agreement was executed on December 20, 2012, almost three years after the complaint was filed. If you are interested in more information about this important case, contact the Department of Justice, Civil Rights Division, ADA Information line at 800-514-0301.

Insight: **Maria Laura Acebal, JD. Board Member and Former CEO,** *Food Allergy & Anaphylaxis Network* **(now FARE -** *Food Allergy Research & Education***)**

My family's introduction to food allergies began with a tiny bite of an orange-colored peanut butter cracker, and ended with a rush to the emergency room where two doses of epinephrine were required to stop our toddler's anaphylactic reaction. Not long after the shock of the diagnosis passed and we got used to our "new normal" of reading every single food ingredient label and being perpetually in possession of two epinephrine auto-injectors, I had the thought - a crazy thought, perhaps, since my daughter was only two-years old: "What are we going to do when she has to go away to college?"

Now, having had the opportunity over the last ten years to speak with hundreds of food allergy parents across the country, I know that wasn't such a crazy thought – many of us worry about facing the college milestone when our kids will have to manage their food allergies alone and away from home. How will they be safe?

The Lesley University Settlement Agreement provides us with some important answers about the kind of support that college students with food allergies may expect to receive under the protections provided by the Americans with Disabilities Act (ADA). As such, it is groundbreaking, but not necessarily for the reasons you may think....

Notably, the Lesley University Agreement is the first – and so far the only – look at the ADA in action in the context of food allergies for students at the college level. News of the settlement made a big impact on the food allergy community and many colleges and universities took the opportunity to take stock of their own practices around managing students' food allergies. However, from a legal standpoint, the settlement's reach is very limited. Indeed, it has no precedential value at all: it doesn't have the force of law and is not binding on any other institution. To understand why, let's take a closer look at the ADA and how it is enforced by the U.S. Department of Justice (DOJ).

As we know, Title III of the ADA protects people with disabilities from discrimination in places of public accommodation, including private institutions of higher learning. Violators of Title III may be subject to civil penalties of $55,000 for the first violation and $110,000 for any subsequent violations. The process of enforcing the ADA begins when an individual files a written complaint with DOJ's Disability Rights Section. Attorneys at the Disability Rights Section then have the job of investigating the allegations in the complaint and deciding among three possible courses of action: negotiating a settlement without involving the courts; filing a lawsuit if attempts at settlement have failed; or, dropping the matter entirely.

In the Lesley University case, a negotiated settlement was reached: a legal contract was signed between Lesley University and DOJ wherein Lesley University agreed to perform very specific actions enumerated in the agreement. Under contract law, of course, these promised actions are binding only on the parties to the contract; they impose no legal requirements on any other person or institution not a signatory to the agreement. Moreover, no court of law has even had occasion to see the settlement agreement, and most likely won't, unless Lesley University fails to comply with the terms and DOJ files a lawsuit for breach of contract. So, what does this mean? Is the Lesley University case not at all important? No, far from it. As food allergy families will gratefully recognize, the breadth of the requirements included in the settlement show a deep understanding of the realities of living with food allergies. (One of my favorites is the required training - every semester - for all food service staff.) Thus, though we can't cite the Lesley University settlement as binding legal authority, we can take comfort in the fact that the enforcers of the ADA at DOJ really "get it" – no small thing for all of us who love someone with food allergies.

The Food Allergen Labeling and Consumer Protection Act

The Food Allergen Labeling and Consumer Protection Act (FALCPA) adopted in 2006, requires that food sold within the U.S. which contains a "major food allergen", defined as one of *"the Big Eight"*, must be listed on the product's label in plain language. *Foods that are not included in "the Big Eight", however, do not have to be specifically declared. F*or example, sesame and garlic might be foods included in "natural flavors" found in an ingredient list, however they might not be clearly identified by name. In addition, FALCPA does not regulate allergen advisory labels on packages, but rather instructs manufacturers to be truthful in what is printed. A study investigating possible ambiguities with advisory labeling found that a total of 25 different types of advisory language exist, a fact that presents a definite challenge for the food-allergic consumer.

U.S. Food and Drug Administration Food Code 2013

While food service operations in public schools have a *specific* regulatory code, university dining services do not. They are, however, subject to general regulatory codes applicable to all establishments that serve food. U.S. Food Code 2013 is an example of this. According to the U.S. Food and Drug Administration, "It represents FDA's best advice for a uniform system of provisions that address the safety and protection of food offered at retail and in food service." Section 2-102.11 of Food Code 2013 states that a food-service manager should be present whenever food is being served, and that this person must be knowledgeable about food allergies, including cleaning protocols to avoid cross-contact, and in the recognition of an allergic reaction. Food Code 2103 also requires food allergy education and training for food service employees as it relates to their specific job responsibilities.

TAKE AWAY NOTES

➢ The Americans with Disabilities Act of 1990 (ADA) and Section 504 of the Rehabilitation Act of 1973, are both federal disability laws written to protect the rights of individuals with disabilities.

➢ Most public and private universities in the United States are subject to the requirements of the ADA and/or Section 504. This means they must provide *reasonable* accommodations which would allow their disabled students to participate safely and enjoy the same educational benefits as nondisabled students.

➢ The Office for Civil Rights (OCR), within the United States Department of Education, recognizes ***allergy*** as a "hidden disability."

➢ The ADA Amendments Act of 2008 broadened the meaning of disability to include eating and conditions that are episodic, such as an anaphylactic reaction.

- ➢ As a result of the judgment in the Lesley University settlement agreement (DJ 202-36-231), food allergies may constitute a disability under the ADA, 42 U.S.C. § 12102.

- ➢ It is the student's responsibility to initiate the process with the college or university's Disability Services Office, and to provide written documentation of the disability from a physician or other professional.

CHAPTER FIVE

Food Allergies: A Refresher

"The goal of education is the advancement of knowledge and the dissemination of truth."

-John F. Kennedy

Many of you reading this book have been managing a food allergy, or multiple food allergies and food intolerances, for what may seem like an eternity. You have learned a lot, of that I am certain. This chapter is intended to confirm what you know, and answer questions about information you may have forgotten. You may even learn something that you didn't know before!

For the newly diagnosed, you are in the learning phase, and most likely trying to gather the facts and make some sense out of what having a food allergy will mean. For you, the information in this chapter is an overview of an important collection of key facts related to food allergy. This will be a good resource to use as a referral, when you need it.

The goal: to make this college journey a safe one!

FOOD ALLERGY

Food allergy is defined by the National Institute of Allergy and Infectious Diseases (NIAID) as: "an adverse health effect arising from a specific immune response that occurs reproducibly on exposure to a given food." In plain language, food allergy is an abnormal response of the body's immune system to specific food proteins. For a person with this diagnosis, the immune system, in essence, misreads the information it receives, and mistakenly identifies the protein in the food to which the person is allergic as being harmful. When a person is re-exposed to this offending food, an allergic reaction will be triggered.

A FOOD INTOLERANCE

For people who have a **food intolerance**, as opposed to a true food allergy, the body's immune system is not involved and IgE antibodies are not produced. Rather, this is a metabolic disorder which does not allow the body to properly digest the food being consumed. Lactose intolerance, an example of a food intolerance, occurs when someone is unable to break down lactose, which is a sugar present in milk products. For these individuals, exposure to milk will most likely cause considerable discomfort, such as an upset stomach, abdominal bloating and other gastrointestinal symptoms.

CELIAC DISEASE

Celiac disease is an inherited, autoimmune disease. It causes problems with the body's response to gluten, a protein found in wheat, barley, rye and triticale, and doesn't allow for the lining of the small intestine (the villi) to properly absorb nutrients from food. Symptoms of celiac disease are chronic, and may include stomach bloating, abdominal pain, vomiting, diarrhea, constipation and weight loss. These symptoms are unlike symptoms of a food allergic reaction and anaphylaxis, because they do not appear in a rapid and acute way. Strict avoidance of foods that contain gluten is required to manage these chronic and uncomfortable symptoms. The National Institutes of Health (NIH) estimates that one in 141 Americans has celiac disease.

SYMPTOMS OF ALLERGIC REACTIONS

There are many different symptoms that may occur when a person with a food allergy is exposed to the allergenic food. The symptoms that develop will depend on which body system(s) has become involved. For example, allergen exposure to the **skin** may provoke itchy, red hives, and swelling (edema) of the area of the skin that has come in contact with the allergen, most commonly in the lips, tongue and/or eyelids. Although most allergic reactions begin with skin symptoms, this is not always the case.

When a food allergen reaches the **gastrointestinal system** (stomach and intestines), a person may experience abdominal cramps, gas, nausea, vomiting and diarrhea. If the **respiratory system** is affected, symptoms such as a stuffy or runny nose, sneezing or coughing - often repetitively, and difficulty swallowing, may develop. The person's voice may change from how it normally sounds, and become either high-pitched or lower. Symptoms of asthma, such as wheezing or shortness of breath, may develop. The onset of respiratory symptoms often signals that the allergic reaction is becoming more severe.

When the **cardiovascular system** is involved, the reaction has become severe and is life-threatening. Symptoms may include paleness, a bluish tint of the skin, dizziness, feeling faint, confusion and/or a drop in blood pressure. People who have experienced these types of symptoms have described feeling a profound sense of impending doom.

SYMPTOMS OF AN ALLERGIC REACTION

Skin
Hives
Swelling of the Affected Area (often the lips, tongue, eyelids)
Itchy, Red Rash (Eczema Flare)

Gastrointestinal

Cramps	Diarrhea
Nausea	Vomiting

Respiratory

Itchy, watery eyes	Difficulty Swallowing	Coughing
Runny or Stuffy Nose	Tightness in the Chest	Shortness of Breath
Sneezing (often repetitive)	Wheezing	Change in Voice

Cardiovascular

Dizziness	Skin turns Pale or Bluish
Confusion	Chest Pain
Feeling Faint, Weak	Drop in Blood Pressure

Anaphylaxis

The most severe form of an allergic reaction is called "anaphylaxis." Anaphylaxis is defined as:

"Anaphylaxis is a serious allergic reaction that is rapid in onset and may cause death."

The symptoms of an anaphylactic reaction usually appear within five to 30 minutes after someone has been exposed to their allergen. It is possible for symptoms of an anaphylactic reaction to subside after treatment, only to reappear with a vengeance, most typically four to eight hours later. This is referred to as a biphasic reaction and statistically, 5-20% of all cases of anaphylaxis are biphasic.

It's important to keep in mind that allergic reactions may vary from episode to episode, and from person to person. While one reaction may be mild, the next reaction might be severe and life-threatening. Symptoms may start off very mild in nature but could progress to a severe reaction very rapidly, sometimes within minutes. Unfortunately, there is no way to predict which symptoms will develop after exposure to an offending allergen, or how severe or mild the reaction will be. (Diagnostic Criteria for Anaphylaxis is included in *Supplemental Materials* found at the end of this chapter.)

Risk Factors for Anaphylaxis

► A Previous History of Anaphylaxis   ► Peanut or Tree Nut Allergy

► Delay in Treating with Epinephrine   ► Asthma

► The Teenage Years

You Should Know:

► It is possible to experience anaphylaxis without having any hives.

► Strict avoidance of the allergenic food(s) is the ONLY way to prevent an allergic reaction and anaphylaxis.

FOODS RESPONSIBLE FOR ALLERGIC REACTIONS

Any food to which a person is allergic is capable of causing symptoms of an allergic reaction. There are eight foods, however, which are commonly referred to as **"the Top Eight"** because they are primarily responsible for causing the majority of allergic reactions to food in the U.S. They are: **peanuts, tree nuts, milk, eggs, wheat, soy, fish and shellfish**. Seed allergies are becoming much more prevalent, and include such foods as sesame, poppy, sunflower, mustard and cottonseed allergies. *More than 170 foods have been reported to cause symptoms of an allergic reaction.*

HOW YOU CAN BE EXPOSED TO A FOOD ALLERGEN

There are four ways in which people with food allergies may be exposed to one of their food allergens. It is important to understand there are different risks associated with each route of exposure.

Ingestion: Eating a food to which we are allergic will undoubtedly trigger symptoms of an allergic reaction. It's important to understand that eating even just an infinitesimal amount of the allergenic food can cause symptoms of an allergic reaction. Successfully avoiding food allergens requires constant effort and relentless ingredient label reading.

Skin Contact: An allergic reaction may occur when the allergen comes into contact with a person's skin. An exposure of this type may produce only skin symptoms, such as hives, redness and localized swelling. Allergic reactions of this nature are usually relatively mild. It is possible, however, to be unaware that the skin has come into contact with the food allergen, because it may be too small to be visible. The risk here is that the allergen then may be inadvertently transferred from the hands to the eyes, nose and/or mouth. When this happens, the allergen has now entered the person's body through the mucous membranes, and this scenario could initiate a systemic, and more serious, allergic reaction.

Example: Skin contact with a food allergen can happen when touching a table surface in the dining hall, or common area that has not been cleaned properly or regularly. Food residue on surfaces is not always visible, and consequently, can be difficult to purposefully avoid.

Inhalation: It is possible for tiny particles of a food to be released into the air and become airborne. If these particles were inhaled by a student who is allergic to the food, it is possible that student would experience an allergic reaction through what is called "inhalation exposure". Symptoms resulting from inhalation are typically itchy eyes, runny nose, sneezing or coughing, similar to allergic symptoms from other airborne allergens, such as dust, pollen or animal dander. These symptoms can be mild, though in some instances, inhalation exposure can cause a more serious allergic reaction.

Example: Inhalation exposure may occur when boiling or steaming foods, such as milk or fish, or even brewing hazelnut coffee, for example. These processes will release the protein of that food into the air, and these particles will not necessarily be visible. Similarly, this process can also happen when an allergic individual is near foods such as peanuts or nuts being eaten, particularly if they are being shelled at the same time. Science experiments that cook or heat a food in an effort to analyze its properties also could be problematic for the student allergic to the food being studied.

Cross-Contact: When one food comes into contact with another food, the proteins of each food will inevitably mix (until recently, this process was referred to as cross-contamination). When this happens, each food will then contain small amounts of the other food, although the presence of both foods may be invisible to the observer.

Example: Cross-contact is a concern in a college or university dining hall in several possible scenarios. If during food preparation, one food is being prepared on a counter, and prior to cleaning, another food is prepared on the same area of the counter, cross-contact of the foods is very likely. When cooking utensils are not cleaned between handling different foods, then again, cross-contact of the foods will occur. If serious precautions are not followed, salad and food bars present multiple risks for the cross-contact of foods.

TREATMENT

Epinephrine is the ONLY medicine capable of reversing the symptoms of anaphylaxis. It is most effective when given as soon as the symptoms of anaphylaxis have been recognized. Epinephrine is available with a prescription, and everyone who is diagnosed with a life-threatening food allergy should carry an epinephrine auto-injector with them *at all times*.

At the date of this book's publication, there is more than one choice of auto-injector available with a prescription. The device most people are familiar with is the **EpiPen®** made by Mylan Specialty L.P. It is available in two strengths, either 0.15mg or 0.3mg, and is packaged as a double-pack. There are step-by-step instructions written on the device to guide people in its use. You should be aware that in 2016, Mylan adjusted the hold time needed for the EpiPen® and the EpiPen Jr.® during the delivery of the medicine from ten seconds to just three seconds. In addition to the EpiPen®, Mylan announced in late August, 2016, its plan to launch its first generic epinephrine auto-injector to the EpiPen®. According to the Mylan website, this generic device is expected to be available within several weeks of this notification, and will be sold as a two-pack in both 0.15mg and 0.3mg. It will be discounted 50% as compared to the EpiPen®. For more information about how to administer the EpiPen®, you can go to: https://www.epipen.com/about-epipen/how-to-use-epipen.

A second choice is a **generic** device sold under the name "epinephrine injection, USP auto-injector," which is manufactured by Impax Laboratories, Inc. This auto-injector is available in 0.15mg or 0.3mg, and is only packaged as a twin-pack.

Please be aware that each brand of epinephrine auto-injector device will have different instructions for its use, so it's important to be familiar with the instructions for the device you choose to carry. You should also be aware that the generic epinephrine injection, USP auto-injector cannot be substituted for the EpiPen® or the EpiPen Jr.®. In other words, if your physician writes a prescription for the EpiPen®, your pharmacist may not substitute this and instead give you the generic epinephrine injection, USP auto-injector.

> ***You Should Know***:**Auvi-Q®**, an auto-injector device manufactured by Sanofi-Aventis U.S. LLC, was voluntarily recalled in October, 2015, due to the potential for inaccurate delivery of the correct dosage. Sanofi US announced on February 23, 2016, that the license and development agreement between Sanofi and kaléo Inc. (the developer of Auvi-Q®), will end later this year. Future plans by kaléo Inc. to bring Auvi-Q® back to the market are being evaluated by kaléo Inc. (The Auvi-Q® device first

became available in January, 2013, and had several novel features: it was the size of a credit card and shaped like a cell phone; when activated, it had voice instructions, as well as written instructions to guide the user with its administration; delivery of the medicine required five seconds; the needle retracted once the medicine had been delivered.)

Adrenaclick®, an epinephrine auto-injector device formerly manufactured by Lineage Therapeutics, Inc., a subsidiary of Amedra Pharmaceuticals, LLC, is no longer being made. At the time of this book's publication, there are no plans for it to be commercially available in the immediate future, according to a representative of Impax Laboratories, Inc. which acquired both Amedra Pharmaceuticals, LLC and Lineage Therapeutics, Inc.

* The pharmaceutical industry can have what may seem to the consumer to be rapid changes, and product availability may change almost overnight. Check with your health care provider and your pharmacist when you have questions about what epinephrine auto-injector devices are available.

More important reminders: Epinephrine should be administered in the muscle of the outer thigh because that is where the medicine will be absorbed most quickly. It is important to understand that epinephrine should not cause any *serious* side effects in an otherwise healthy, young person. Once someone has been treated with epinephrine, 911 should be called immediately so that emergency medical personnel can respond and transfer the person to the hospital emergency room for observation in case of a biphasic reaction. Having **two** epinephrine auto-injectors on hand *at all times* is a good idea for two reasons:

> 1) as a back-up should anything go wrong during the delivery of the medicine, and

> 2) to use to deliver a second dose of epinephrine if the first dose is ineffective, or if the person were to experience a biphasic reaction. Another important reminder: epinephrine needs to be stored in a temperature-controlled environment, and should not be exposed to temperatures higher than 86 degrees or lower than 59 degrees.

These are the facts. Having the knowledge required to 1.) recognize symptoms of an allergic reaction, and 2.) understand that the symptoms may progress rapidly to anaphylaxis, becomes critical, because it will promote better decision-making in response to this type of an emergency, and help to insure that the appropriate medical intervention will be accessed quickly.

You Should Know:

Anaphylaxis is not a risk for a food intolerance or celiac disease, and because of that, epinephrine is not required to treat the symptoms of either of these health conditions.

TAKE AWAY NOTES

➢ Exposure to *ANY* food you are allergic to is capable of causing symptoms of an allergic reaction.

➢ Strict avoidance of your food allergens is the *ONLY* way to prevent an allergic reaction.

➢ Careful reading of ingredient lists *EVERY* time a product is purchased is needed in order to avoid exposure or accidental ingestion of your food allergen(s).

➢ Anaphylaxis is a life-threatening medical emergency. Make sure you know the possible signs and symptoms of an allergic reaction and anaphylaxis. Prompt treatment with epinephrine is the *ONLY* way to reverse the symptoms of anaphylaxis.

➢ *ALWAYS* carry your prescribed epinephrine auto-injector (preferably two), and know how to use it!

SUPPLEMENTAL MATERIALS

———————————————————

FOOD ALLERGIES: KEY POINTS

There are 17.5 million full and part-time college students in the United States (22% of these students have allergies)

- A true food allergy involves an abnormal response of the immune system and causes the body to produce IgE antibodies to a particular food protein. The most severe form of this reaction is called **anaphylaxis.**
- If not treated promptly, anaphylaxis may result in death.
- Annually in the United States, there are 203,000 hospital emergency room visits for acute food-induced allergic reactions.
- Food-induced anaphylaxis accounts for approximately 150-200 deaths per year.
- Symptoms of an allergic reaction can be caused by as little as 2 milligrams of a peanut (approximately 1/250th of a peanut), for example. The amount of allergen needed to cause a reaction varies from person to person.
- Most food allergic reactions occur from eating an unexpected or hidden ingredient, or unknowingly ingesting the allergen from cross-contact.
- Symptoms of a reaction, such as vomiting, hives or respiratory distress, may vary from person to person.
- Some individuals may develop symptoms of an allergic reaction when the allergen comes in contact with their skin (tactile) OR from inhaling airborne particles of the food protein.
- There is no way to predict how an allergic reaction will develop. Symptoms may progress from mild to severe in several minutes.
- Delay in treatment with epinephrine, asthma, and the teenage years, are considered risk factors for fatal anaphylaxis in food-allergic individuals.
- The incidence of peanut allergy in the U.S. has tripled since 1997.
- A <u>New England Journal of Medicine</u> study found that **four out of six fatalities** from a food allergic reaction **OCCURRED AT SCHOOL**.

AVOIDANCE is the **ONLY** way to prevent accidental ingestion and a possible life-threatening reaction.

Anaphylaxis

"Anaphylaxis is a serious allergic reaction that is rapid in onset and may cause death."

Anaphylaxis is highly likely to occur when any one of the following 3 criteria are met:

1. SKIN SYMPTOMS OR SWOLLEN LIPS AND EITHER:
   a. DIFFICULTY BREATHING **OR**
   b. REDUCED BLOOD PRESSURE

2. AN INDIVIDUAL HAD EXPOSURE TO A "SUSPECTED ALLERGEN"
   AND 2 OR MORE OF THE FOLLOWING OCCUR:
   a. SKIN SYMPTOMS OR SWOLLEN LIPS OR TONGUE
   b. DIFFICULTY BREATHING
   c. REDUCED BLOOD PRESSURE
   d. GASTRO-INTESTINAL SYMPTOMS SUCH AS VOMITTING, DIARRHEA OR CRAMPING

3. AN INDIVIDUAL HAS HAD EXPOSURE TO A "KNOWN ALLERGEN"
   AND EXPERIENCES:
   a. REDUCED BLOOD PRESSURE

(Symptoms may occur within minutes to hours after exposure to the allergen.)

Epinephrine should be given immediately when the above criteria are met _or_ for an individual with a history of life-threatening reactions who has had exposure to an allergen and begins to have symptoms quickly, even if they are mild.

Source: Adapted from the 2nd National Institute of Allergy and Infectious Disease/FAAN Anaphylaxis Symposium July, 2005

"TOP EIGHT" ALLERGENS
OFTEN FOUND IN PREPARED FOODS

Note: This is only a partial list of foods containing the Top Eight allergens.

__MILK__ may be found in the following products:

Cheeses, cottage cheese, butter, margarine, sour cream, whipped cream, ice cream, sweetened condensed milk, evaporated milk, powdered milk, sherbet, hot dogs, deli meats, yogurt, quick breads, gravies, dips, cake mixes, non-dairy creamers, custards, pastries, canned tuna fish, ham, luncheon meats, hot dogs, sausages, pasta dishes, pancakes, waffles, French toast, popsicles, crackers, baby crackers, bread, rolls, Tostito chips® (lime), Cheetos®, pretzels, cookies, chocolate, cereals, microwave popcorn and candies.

"K", "U", "Circle U" = __KOSHER__ label which means that a food has been certified by a rabbi as meeting the Jewish standard for dietary restrictions of milk, meat, and shellfish.

"K-D", "D", or "DE" = the presence of milk protein or foods that were processed on equipment also used for milk products.

"PAREVE" = foods that *usually* do not contain dairy products or meat products.

__EGGS__ may be found in the following products:

glaze on baked goods, pasta, custard bases to ice cream, breads, bagels, cakes and other baked goods, pancakes, waffles, soufflés, French toast, macaroni, mayonnaise, meringue, marshmallows, custards, pretzels, some ice creams, sauces, dressings and pasta dishes, candy, jelly beans, and fried foods from vendors who use same vat for egg-battered foods.

__PEANUTS (also known as goobers, groundnuts, earthnuts)__ may be found in the following products:

Peanut oil, peanut butter, peanut flour, chili, brown gravy, spaghetti sauce, barbecue sauce, Satay sauces, egg rolls and other Chinese foods, enchilada sauce, some vegetarian foods, instant rice mixes, cereals, hot cocoa, candy, gourmet popcorn, granola bars, mandelonas (peanuts soaked in almond flavoring), ice creams, some Good Humor™ ice creams, chocolates (cross-contact), M&Ms, gummy bears, jelly beans (especially gourmet brands), snack-size chips and cookies, brownie mix and many pastries and baked goods.

TREE NUTS (almonds, cashews, filberts, hazelnuts, macadamia nuts, chestnuts, mandelonas, pecans, pistachios, walnuts [Black and English], butternuts [a white walnut], pralines, pine nuts [pinon, pignolia, pignoli, Indian nut], brazil nuts and hickory nuts, among others) may be found in the following products:

Nut flours, butters and oils, Nutella® (hazelnut and chocolate), ice cream, yogurt, candies, nougat, cookies, breads, muffins, baked goods, some sauces, salads and salad dressings, pie crusts, barbecue sauce, cereals, granolas, granola bars, pesto, marzipan (almond paste), cake mixes, brownie mixes, many baked goods and desserts, some cookies, trail and snack mixes, flavored liquors such as amaretto (almond), and Frangelico (hazelnut).

*Both peanuts and tree nuts are often use in beanbags, shampoos, soaps, skin creams, bath oils and cosmetics.
*Coconut may be considered a fruit, nut or seed

WHEAT may be found in the following products:
Breads, pastas, semolina, farina, durum, kamut, triticale, spelt, faro, cereals, muesli, bulgur, couscous, pilafs, seitan, crackers, Matzoh, flour, baked goods, wheat germ oil, ice cream cones, pizza dough.

SOY may be found in the following products:
Soybean oil, soy (also known as "edamame"), soy sauce, margarines, shortenings, tofu, canned tuna, cereals, crackers, many processed meats, and in salad dressings, sauces and soups.

FISH AND SHELLFISH may be found in the following products:
caesar salad, Worcestershire sauce, salad dressing, bouillabaisse, surimi (Alaska Pollock, pacific whiting, imitation crabmeat).

FOODS THAT ARE *NOT* NUTS
nutmeg: seed from tropical tree water chestnut: edible plant root

FARE
Food Allergy Research & Education

FOOD ALLERGY & ANAPHYLAXIS EMERGENCY CARE PLAN

Name: _____ D.O.B.: _____

Allergy to: _____

Weight: _____ lbs. Asthma: [ ] **Yes (higher risk for a severe reaction)** [ ] **No**

PLACE
PICTURE
HERE

NOTE: Do not depend on antihistamines or inhalers (bronchodilators) to treat a severe reaction. USE EPINEPHRINE.

Extremely reactive to the following allergens: _____

THEREFORE:

[ ] If checked, give epinephrine immediately if the allergen was LIKELY eaten, for ANY symptoms.

[ ] If checked, give epinephrine immediately if the allergen was DEFINITELY eaten, even if no symptoms are apparent.

FOR ANY OF THE FOLLOWING:
SEVERE SYMPTOMS

LUNG
Short of breath, wheezing, repetitive cough

HEART
Pale, blue, faint, weak pulse, dizzy

THROAT
Tight, hoarse, trouble breathing/ swallowing

MOUTH
Significant swelling of the tongue and/or lips

SKIN
Many hives over body, widespread redness

GUT
Repetitive vomiting, severe diarrhea

OTHER
Feeling something bad is about to happen, anxiety, confusion

OR A COMBINATION
of symptoms from different body areas.

1. **INJECT EPINEPHRINE IMMEDIATELY.**
2. **Call 911.** Tell emergency dispatcher the person is having anaphylaxis and may need epinephrine when emergency responders arrive.
- Consider giving additional medications following epinephrine:
  » Antihistamine
  » Inhaler (bronchodilator) if wheezing
- Lay the person flat, raise legs and keep warm. If breathing is difficult or they are vomiting, let them sit up or lie on their side.
- If symptoms do not improve, or symptoms return, more doses of epinephrine can be given about 5 minutes or more after the last dose.
- Alert emergency contacts.
- Transport patient to ER, even if symptoms resolve. Patient should remain in ER for at least 4 hours because symptoms may return.

MILD SYMPTOMS

NOSE
Itchy/runny nose, sneezing

MOUTH
Itchy mouth

SKIN
A few hives, mild itch

GUT
Mild nausea/ discomfort

FOR MILD SYMPTOMS FROM MORE THAN ONE SYSTEM AREA, GIVE EPINEPHRINE.

FOR MILD SYMPTOMS FROM A SINGLE SYSTEM AREA, FOLLOW THE DIRECTIONS BELOW:

1. Antihistamines may be given, if ordered by a healthcare provider.
2. Stay with the person; alert emergency contacts.
3. Watch closely for changes. If symptoms worsen, give epinephrine.

MEDICATIONS/DOSES

Epinephrine Brand or Generic: _____

Epinephrine Dose: [ ] 0.15 mg IM [ ] 0.3 mg IM

Antihistamine Brand or Generic: _____

Antihistamine Dose: _____

Other (e.g., inhaler-bronchodilator if wheezing): _____

_____

_____

PATIENT OR PARENT/GUARDIAN AUTHORIZATION SIGNATURE   DATE   PHYSICIAN/HCP AUTHORIZATION SIGNATURE   DATE

FORM PROVIDED COURTESY OF FOOD ALLERGY RESEARCH & EDUCATION (FARE) (FOODALLERGY.ORG) 7/2016

© 2016, Food Allergy Research & Education.
Used with permission.

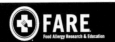 **FARE** Food Allergy Research & Education | **FOOD ALLERGY & ANAPHYLAXIS EMERGENCY CARE PLAN**

EPIPEN® AUTO-INJECTOR DIRECTIONS

1. Remove the EpiPen Auto-Injector from the clear carrier tube.
2. Remove the blue safety release by pulling straight up without bending or twisting it.
3. Swing and firmly push orange tip against mid-outer thigh until it 'clicks'.
4. Hold firmly in place for 3 seconds (count slowly 1, 2, 3).
5. Remove auto-injector from the thigh and massage the injection area for 10 seconds.

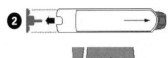
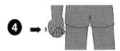

ADRENACLICK® (EPINEPHRINE INJECTION, USP) AUTO-INJECTOR DIRECTIONS

1. Remove the outer case.
2. Remove grey caps labeled "1" and "2".
3. Place red rounded tip against mid-outer thigh.
4. Press down hard until needle enters thigh.
5. Hold in place for 10 seconds. Remove from thigh.

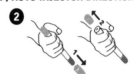
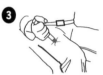

ADMINISTRATION AND SAFETY INFORMATION FOR ALL AUTO-INJECTORS:

1. Do not put your thumb, fingers or hand over the tip of the auto-injector or inject into any body part other than mid-outer thigh. In case of accidental injection, go immediately to the nearest emergency room.
2. If administering to a young child, hold their leg firmly in place before and during injection to prevent injuries.
3. Epinephrine can be injected through clothing if needed.
4. Call 911 immediately after injection.

OTHER DIRECTIONS/INFORMATION (may self-carry epinephrine, may self-administer epinephrine, etc.):

Treat the person before calling emergency contacts. The first signs of a reaction can be mild, but symptoms can worsen quickly.

EMERGENCY CONTACTS — CALL 911

RESCUE SQUAD: _____

DOCTOR: _____ PHONE: _____

PARENT/GUARDIAN: _____ PHONE: _____

OTHER EMERGENCY CONTACTS

NAME/RELATIONSHIP: _____

PHONE: _____

NAME/RELATIONSHIP: _____

PHONE: _____

FORM PROVIDED COURTESY OF FOOD ALLERGY RESEARCH & EDUCATION (FARE) (FOODALLERGY.ORG) 7/2016

GLOSSARY

DEFINITION OF TERMS

Accommodation - is a modification to a service or practice that will allow a student the opportunity to participate safely in the college program, including the ability to have access to safe foods to eat. It refers to the requirements of Section 504 of the Rehabilitation Act of 1973.

Americans with Disabilities Act of 1990 - is a federal civil rights law enforced by the U.S. Department of Justice. This law states that, ". . . no individual shall be discriminated against on the basis of disability in the full and equal enjoyment of the goods, services, facilities, privileges, advantages . . . of any place of public accommodation . . . ."

The ADA Amendments Act of 2008 (ADAAA) - went into effect on January 1, 2009, and broadened the scope of the interpretation of the definition of disability. The amendments expanded the definition of major life activities to include eating, and to include conditions that are episodic.

Anaphylaxis - is a serious allergic reaction that is rapid in onset and may cause death. Fatal reactions may occur without skin symptoms, such as hives, and any food can be the cause of anaphylaxis. Anaphylaxis presents a life-threatening medical emergency and immediate medical treatment is required.

Celiac Disease - also called gluten-sensitive enteropathy or sprue, is an inherited, autoimmune disease. It causes problems with the body's response to gluten - a protein found in wheat, barley, rye and triticale, and doesn't allow for the lining of the small intestine (the villi) to properly absorb nutrients from food. Symptoms of celiac disease are chronic and may have many possible symptoms, including stomach bloating, abdominal pain, vomiting, diarrhea, constipation and weight loss.

Cross-Contact - occurs when one food comes into contact with another food, and the proteins of each food mix together. Each food will contain small amounts of the other food, although often this won't be visible.

Disability - is defined as a physical or mental impairment that substantially limits one or more major life activities. A physical or mental impairment is defined as "any physiological disorder or condition . . . affecting one or more body systems".

Emergency Treatment Plan - is the written treatment plan written by a physician/allergist which outlines the steps to follow to treat an allergic reaction and anaphylaxis.

Epinephrine - is the only medication capable of reversing the symptoms of anaphylaxis. It is critical that epinephrine is administered immediately if anaphylaxis is suspected.

Epinephrine Auto-Injector - is a spring-based, self-injectable device that delivers epinephrine when administered. It is designed for people without medical training to treat anaphylaxis.

Food Allergen Labeling and Consumer Protection Act of 2004 (FALCPA) - requires that ingredient labels on food packages list the presence of a "major food allergen", in clear language, if present as an ingredient in the food being sold.

Food Allergy - is an abnormal response of the body's immune system to specific food proteins, resulting in an allergic reaction with re-exposure to the food.

"Major Food Allergens", "Top Eight", "Big Eight" - milk, eggs, peanuts, tree nuts, fish, shellfish, wheat, and soy.

Resident Advisors - college students, typically upperclassmen, who are selected to live in a residence hall and assist students living on their floor. They receive training in building relationships, conflict resolution, and recognition of various issues of concern.

Resident Directors - adult residence staff, usually graduate students or professors, who live in a residence hall and supervise the Resident Advisors assigned to their building.

Section 504 of the Rehabilitation Act of 1973 - is a civil rights law enforced by the Office of Civil Rights (OCR) within the U.S. Department of Education. This federal law is constructed to protect the rights of individuals with a disability and "prohibit discrimination on the basis of disability in education…in any program or institution receiving federal funds . . . ." The OCR recognizes *allergy* as a "hidden disability." Students with physician-documented, life-threatening food allergies are generally considered to have a disability under this law.

REFERENCES

American Academy of Allergy and Asthma Immunologists, *"Off to College with Allergies and Asthma." www.AAAAI.org.* PDF Fact Sheet.

Bock SA, Munoz-Furlong A, Sampson HA. "Further fatalities caused by anaphylactic reactions to food, 2001-6." Letter to Editor. *J Allergy Clin Immunol* 2007; 119: 1016-18.

Boyce, JA., et al. "Guidelines for the diagnosis and management of food allergy in the United States: Report of the NIAID-sponsored expert panel." *J Allergy Clin Immunol* 2010; 126:S1-S58.

"Checklist for College with Food Allergies." by Nicole Smith, posted online, April 16, 2014. www.allergicchild.com/checklist-for-college-with-food-allergies/.

Choi JH, Rajagopal L. "Food allergy knowledge, attitudes, practices, and training of foodservice workers at a university foodservice operation in the Midwestern United States." Elsevier, *Food Control* 2013; 31 (2): 474-481.

Clark S, et al. "Frequency of US emergency department visits for food-related acute allergic reactions." *J Allergy Clin Immunol* 2011; 127 (3): 682-3.

Costa DJ, et al. "Guidelines for allergic rhinitis to be used in primary care." *Prim Care Respir J* 2009; 18 (4): 258-265.

Cummings AJ, et al. "The psychosocial impact of food allergy and food hypersensitivity in children, adolescents and their families: a review." *Allergy* 2010; 65(8): 933-945.

Food Allergen Labeling and Consumer Protection Act of 2004 (FALCPA), 108-282, §201, 118 Stat.905 (2004).

"Going to College with Food Allergies: An Interview with North Carolina State's Registered Dietitian." Interview with Lisa Eberhart, RD, Director of Nutrition and Wellness, posted in www.PeanutAllergy.com.

Greenhawt MJ, Singer AM, Baptist AP. "Food allergy and food allergy attitudes among college students." *J Allergy Clin Immunol* 2009; 124: 323-7.

Hallett R, Teuber SS. "Kissing and Food Reactions." Letter to the Editor. *N Engl J Med* 2002; 347: 1210.

Herbert LJ, Dalquist LM. "Perceived history of anaphylaxis and parental overprotection, autonomy, anxiety, and depression in food allergic young adults." *J Clin Psychol Med Settings* 2008; 15 (4): 261-269.

"How to Survive Commons with a Food Allergy." Article by Jeffrey Careyva, *The Daily Pennsylvanian,* October 26, 2015.

"*Joint Guidance on the Application of the Family Educational Rights and Privacy Act (FERPA) and the Health Insurance Portability and Accountability Act of 1996 (HIPAA) to Student Health Records.*" U.S. Department of Health and Human Services and U.S. Department of Education, November, 2008.

LeBovidge JS, Strauch H, Kalish LA, Schneider LC. "Assessment of psychological distress among children and adolescents with food allergy." *J Allergy Clin Immunol* 2009; 124: 122-8.

Lyons AC, Forde EM. "Food allergy in young adults: perceptions and psychological effects." *J Health Psych* 2004; 9 (4): 497-504.

Maloney JM, et al. "Peanut allergen exposure through saliva: Assessments and interventions to reduce exposure." *J Allergy Clin Immunol* 2006; 118: 719-24.

"Managing Food Allergies in a Campus Setting." Article by Beth Winthrop, MS, RD, CNSC, *Tastings*, Fall, 2013, newsletter for *Food & Culinary Professionals.*

"Managing your food allergies in dining halls and dorm rooms." Article by Sloane Miller, *The Washington Post*, September 9, 2011.

Monaco, MA, Rajagopal, L., Bernstein, AL (2012, July). "Experiences of food allergy sufferers with College and University dining Services." Poster presented at the 2012 International Association of Food Protection, July 22-25 in Providence, RI.

Mylan Survey, released 2013. "Parent/Caregiver communications with children/teens/young adults with severe allergies and dating precautions."

Panzer, Rebecca, MA, RD, LD. "Navigating the Gluten Free Diet in College." Guide. www.beyondceliac.org.

Rajagopal, L, Strohbehn CH. "Views of College and University Directors on Food Allergen Policies and Practices in Higher Education Settings." *Journal of Foodservice Management and Education* 2011; 5 (1): 15-21.

Resnick ES, Pieretti MM, Maloney J, Noone S, Munoz-Furlong A, Sicherer SH. "Development of a questionnaire to measure quality of life in adolescents with food allergy: the FAQL-teen." *Ann Allergy Asthma Immunol* 2010; 105 (5): 364-68.

Sampson HA, et al. "Food Allergy: A practice parameter update – 2014. Joint Task Force on Practice Parameters." *J Allergy Clin Immunol* 2014; 134 (5): 1016-25.

Samspon HA, et al. "Second symposium on the definition and management of anaphylaxis: Summary report - second National Institute of Allergy and Infectious Disease/Food Allergy and Anaphylaxis Network symposium." *J Allergy Clin Immunol* 2006; 117: 391-7.

Sampson MA, Munoz-Furlong A, Sicherer SH. "Risk-taking and coping strategies of adolescents and young adults with food allergy." *J Allergy Clin Immunol* 2006; 117; 1440-5.

Shemesh E., et al. "Child and parental reports of bullying in a consecutive sample of children with food allergy." *Pediatrics* 2013; 131: e10-17.

"Student Health: Peanut allergy risk factors on campus and in the dining hall." Article by Alana Joli Abbott, September 3, 2013, posted in www.cengagebrain.com.

"Surviving College with Food Allergies", article by Kristin Musulin, *USA Today*: February 21, 2014.

"The Civil Rights of Students with Hidden Disabilities Under Section 504 of the Rehabilitation Act of 1973." www2.ed.gov/offices/list/ocr/docs.

Trotch, Claudia, "Food For Thought: Applying the ADA to Students with Food Allergies." NACUANOTES, August 27 2014; Vol. 12, No. 7.

United States Department of Justice, Civil Rights Division, article: "Questions and Answers About the Lesley University Agreement and Potential Implications for Individuals with Food Allergies." www.ada.gov/q&a_lesley_university.htm.

United States Department of Justice, Office for Public Affairs, "Justice Department and Lesley University Sign Agreement to Ensure Meal Plan is Inclusive of Students with Celiac Disease and Food Allergies." Released December 20, 2012. www.justice.gov. Justice News.

United States Food and Drug Administration, Food Code 2013. www.fda.gov/downloads/food/guidanceregulation/retailfoodprotection/foodcode/ucm374510.pdf

"Update on Anaphylaxis: Recognition and Treatment in a College Health Service." PowerPoint by Eleanor W. Davidson MD, Sara H. Lee MD. February 27, 2014. *American College Health Association.*

LIST OF RECOMMENDED RESOURCES

Allergic Living Magazine
PO Box 1042
Niagara Falls, New York 14304
888-771-7747
www.allergicliving.com

> *College and Food Allergies Resource Hub*
>
> *"Off to College with Food Allergies and Celiac Disease." Article by Patrick Bennett, Special Report*
>
> *"College with Food Allergies: Lessons From a Seasoned Mom." Article by Nicole Smith*

Allergy & Asthma Network, Mothers of Asthmatics (AANMA)
8229 Boone Boulevard, Suite 260
Vienna, Virginia 22182
800-878-4403
www.allergyasthmanetwork.org

> *"The College Experience: Raising Awareness of Food Allergies on Campus." Article*

AllerTrain™ by MenuTrinfo®
155 North College Avenue, Suite 200
Fort Collins, CO 80524
970-295-4370
www.allertrain.com

> Food Allergy & Gluten Free Training Courses: AllerTrain U *and* AllerTrain RA

American Academy of Asthma, Allergy and Immunology (AAAAI)
555 East Wells Street, Suite 1100
Milwaukee, WI 53202
414-272-6071
www.aaaai.org

> *"Off to College with Allergies and Asthma."* AAAAI, Fact Sheet

American Bar Association
www.americanbar.org.
Services Hotline: 1-800-285-2221

American College Health Association (ACHA)
1362 Mellon Road, Suite 180
Hanover, Maryland 21076
410-859-1500
www.acha.org

American College of Asthma, Allergy and Immunology (ACAAI)
85 W. Algonquin Road, Suite 550
Arlington Heights, IL 60005
847-427-1200
www.acaai.org

> *"Are Your Allergies and Asthma Ready For College?"* ACAAI,
> Information Sheet

American Partnership for Eosinophilic Disorders (APFED)
PO Box 29545
Atlanta, Georgia, 30359
713-493-7749
www.apfed.org

Association on Higher Education and Disability® (AHEAD)
107 Commerce Center Drive, Suite 204
Huntersville, North Carolina 28078
704-947-7779
www.ahead.org

Asthma and Allergy Foundation of America (AAFA)
8201 Corporate Drive, Suite 1000
Landover, Maryland 20785
800-727-8462
www.aafa.org

Asthma and Allergy Foundation of America, New England Chapter
109 Highland Avenue
Needham, MA 02494
781-444-7778
www.asthmaandallergies.org

>   *"Food Allergy and College: Planning for Campus Life" Booklet*
>
>   *"Asthma and Allergies Go to College" Tips*

Beyond Celiac (National Foundation for Celiac Awareness - NFCA)
PO Box 544
Amber, Pennsylvania 19002
844-856-6692
www.beyondceliac.org

>   *"Gluten-Free In College" Toolkit*
>
>   *"Navigating the Gluten Free Diet in College" Guide*

Celiac Disease Foundation
20350 Ventura Boulevard, Suite 240
Woodland Hills, California 91364
818-716-1513
www.celiac.org

Centers for Disease Control and Prevention
Division of Adolescent and School Health
4770 Buford Highway, NE
MS K29
Atlanta, Georgia 30341
800-232-4636
www.cdc.gov

Donahue, Jack, *Gluten-Free University: Survival Guide to College with Food Allergies*. GfreeGuy.com, June, 2015 (Kindle).

Educating For Food Allergies, LLC (EFFA)
80 Washington Street, Building O-53
Norwell, MA 02061
781-982-7029
www.foodallergyed.com

Food Allergy & Anaphylaxis Connection Team (FAACT)
PO Box 511
West Chester, Ohio 45071
513-342-1293
www.foodallergyawarenes.org

Food Allergy Research and Education (FARE)
795 Jones Branch Drive, Suite 1100
McLean, Virginia 22102
800-929-4040
www.foodallergy.org/collegeprogram

> *College Food Allergy Program*
>
> *"A Prospective Student's Guide"*
>
> *"A Current Student's Guide"*
>
> *FARE College Food Allergy Support Group on Facebook*

Gluten Free and More
535 Connecticut Avenue
Norwalk, Connecticut 06856
800-474-8614
www.glutenfreeandmore.com

Kids with Food Allergies – A Division of the Asthma and Allergy Foundation of America
5049 Swamp Road, Suite 303
PO Box 554
Fountainville, Pennsylvania 18923
215-340-7674
www.kidswithfoodallergies.org

Miller, Sloane, *Allergic Girl: Adventures in Living Well with Food Allergies*. Wiley and Sons, Inc., Hoboken, NJ 2011.

Mothers of Children Having Allergies (MOCHA)
www.mochallergies.org

National Association of College and University Food Services (NACUFS)
2525 Jolly Road, Suite 280
Okemos, MI 48864
517-332-2494
www.nacufs.org

National Association of College and University Residence Halls (NACURH)
1115 North 16th Street
Lincoln, Nebraska 68588
424-262-2874
www.nacurh.org

Reino, Jessica, *Food Allergies: The Ultimate Teen Guide (It Happened To Me)*. Rowman & Littlefield Publishers Group, Inc., 4501 Forbes Boulevard, Suite 200, Lanham, Maryland 20706, June, 2015.

Roth, Lily, *Food Allergy Survival Guide, College Edition.* Online publication. www.foodallergysurvivalguide.weebly.com.

Stavola, Elisa, *Living With Life Threatening Food Allergies: A Teenager's Guide To Doing It Well.* CreateSpace Independent Publishing, January, 2015.

The Council of Parent Advocates and Attorneys (COPAA)
PO Box 6767
Towson, Maryland 21285
844-426-7224
www.copaa.org

The International Association of Food Protection (IAFP)
6200 Aurora Avenue, Suite 200W
Des Moines, Iowa 50322
800-369-6337
www.foodprotection.org

United States Department of Education, Office for Civil Rights
Customer Service Team
400 Maryland Avenue, SW
Washington, DC 20202
800-421-3481
www2.ed.gov

> *"Students with Disabilities Preparing for Postsecondary Education:Know Your Rights and Responsibilities."* Pamphlet
>
> *"The Civil Rights of Students with Hidden Disabilities Under Section 504 of the Rehabilitation Act of 1973"*

United States Department of Justice (DOJ), Civil Rights Division
950 Pennsylvania Avenue
Washington, DC 20530
202-514-2000
www.justice.gov

> *"Questions and Answers About the Lesley University Agreement and Potential Implications for Individuals with Food Allergies"*
> www.ada.gov/q&a_lesley_university.htm.
>
> DOJ Americans With Disabilities Act Information Line
> 800-514-0301 (All calls are confidential)
> www.ada.gov/inforline.htm.

United States Food and Drug Administration
10903 New Hampshire Avenue
Silver Spring, Maryland 20993
888-463-6332
www.fda.gov

> Food Code 2013
> (www.fda.gov/downloads/food/guidanceregulation/retailfoodprote ction/foodcode/ucm374510.pdf)

ONLINE RESOURCES

AllergyEats, Guide for food allergy-friendly restaurants in the U.S., www.allergyeats.com

FoodASC, Online directory for the food allergy and sensitivity communities that features resources in a variety of categories, www.foodasc.com

Freedible, Recipes, blogs, conversations, www.freedible.com

Mylan Specialty L.P., "Get Schooled in Anaphylaxis", www.anaphylaxis101.com

SnackSafely, Information for people with food allergies in the U.S., www.snacksafely.com

****

ABOUT THE AUTHOR

Jan Hanson, M.A., is a nationally recognized food allergy educator, author and speaker and has more than 25 years of experience in the area of food allergy management. She is committed to empowering everyone who has a food allergy to live safely and fully. She conducted her first educational workshop to school personnel in 1996, and in 2001, she founded her consulting company, Educating For Food Allergies, LLC (EFFA). She provides guidance in the development of accommodations for use in 504 Plans and Individual Healthcare Plans, and in the writing of school district food allergy management policy. Her company is a registered provider of Professional Development Points with the Massachusetts Department of Education, and also meets the requirements of the Massachusetts Board of Registration in Nursing to provide Contact Hours for Massachusetts school nurses. She has testified in support of legislation in Massachusetts that called for emergency personnel to carry and administer epinephrine, and for food service personnel to be knowledgeable in food allergy issues.

Ms. Hanson is also a former college administrator. After having earned her B.A. in Psychology at Mount Holyoke College, and prior to her involvement as a food allergy educator, Jan earned her Master's Degree in Higher Education Administration from Boston College, and worked as the Assistant Director of Residence at Simmons College. This position required her to live on the residence campus, train and work with Resident Advisors and Resident Directors, and gave her the invaluable experience of interacting with college students on a day-to-day basis, in a very real and personal way.

Jan is the author of the book, *Food Allergies: A Recipe For Success At School*, published in 2012, which has received national recognition and praise, including in *The Washington Post*. She has written numerous articles on the subject of food allergy management published in print and online magazines and newspapers throughout the country, and has been utilized as an expert on this topic by both radio and print journalists, including in the *Miami Herald* and *Allergic Living Magazine.*

Jan was a speaker at the May, 2016 national *Food Allergy Research and Education Conference* (FARE) in Orlando on "Planning For College with Food Allergies", and at the first national FARE Conference in Chicago, June, 2014. She presented at the *4ᵗʰ Annual Utah Food Allergy*

Conference in November, 2014, and she served on two panels at the *Food Allergy Bloggers Conference* held in Las Vegas in November, 2013, and in September, 2014. She presented at the *Visions of Community 2013 Conference* sponsored by the Federation for Children with Special Needs in Boston, and at the 10th Annual *Food Safety Education Conference* hosted by the University of Rhode Island. Jan is a Board Member of the New England Chapter of the Asthma and Allergy Foundation of America.

Ms. Hanson is the proud mother of two sons, who happen to have food allergies, and who graduated from college in 2009 and 2013.

Made in the USA
San Bernardino, CA
13 November 2016